YOGA EMOTIONAL DICTIONARY

Mary Jane Fox

2020

Table of Contents

INTRODUCTION

As much as you might not have any desire to hear if you are run by your brain as opposed to you running it. Well saying this doesn't imply that you have no control and state over your daily, week by week, month to month, yearly and life existence, because obviously, you do have a state in it. Be that as it may, if we are talking rate in control, you consciously versus your unconscious (which you have no conscious control over*) I'm afraid we as a whole come a dismal second. Presently as your indignation maybe arises and you are forming contentions in your mind that you are in full control, stop a moment and think about that reaction. Or then again if you like reveal to me the amount you are consciously mindful of virtually the entirety of your incredibly unpredictable life functions which are going on right now and controlled by your unconscious. Digestion and distribution of nutrients, oxygen exchange and evacuation of contaminations, blood replacement, lymphatic system, skin repair, liver and kidney function, blood pH balance, control over the working of a vast number of muscles moves every day controlling each small movement you make. Do I need to go on? No, you are not in control of most by far of what your body and mind do. Your brain is running you. The brain's control of us in those areas is highly desirable; however, for a great many people there is likewise an absence of authority in progressively close to home behavior areas, and these should concern you. Have you at any point lost your temper and thought twice about it? Of course, you have. That is a case of not being in control of an emotional reaction that you ought to have control over, and it should concern you that you are being run (you did not consciously control your opinion) by your brain.

Presently let's take a gander at this as it applies to a few areas in golf and why you ought to deal with your emotional reactions if you wish to play better. You play a terrible shot and immediately get a little humiliated/irritated/cross/fuming frantic. None of which are useful to you in playing your next shot. I'm sure you comprehend that best performance originates from a casual, quiet mind that is confident and committed to each shot. So it pursues that any negative emotion from shame to humiliation to disturbance or outright fuming displeasure is going to be hurtful to your following chances. The descending spiral is currently gotten underway since you are bound to play awful shots as a result of your poor emotional state, and those awesome shots get you significantly progressively annoyed, right? If you have not experienced this then either you are a Zen Master or from a different planet to us people. I guess you could likewise be extremely fortunate and have no ego which would genuinely help in controlling emotions. I hope you would now be able to see the connection between going into a psychological state that is terrible for playing golf and my earlier claim that you have less control over yourself than you think. If you are totally in control of your emotions then you will never get irritated, cross, furious, humiliated or downright humiliated on the course until kingdom come, since you realize it will compound the situation. The incredible test is not to be in control of our golf game, yet to be in control of our emotions and state of mind, for that is the whole legislative head of performance. While I don't know that you will ever totally master your emotional control when faced with any situation, (and I'm not saying you won't) you can get, genuinely adept at controlling emotions regardless of what you are faced with. There are valid justifications we respond ineffectively to shots on the course, and it boils down to your ego in the end. The universe of contemporary sport psychology has now got various highly effective apparatuses for emotional control ranging from Hypnosis to Cognitive Behavioral Techniques and in particular NLP. (Neuro Linguistic Programming) Sports psychology has progressed enormously just over the most recent ten years, and we have gotten familiar with the human brain function and behavior in that brief span than in all of history.

CHAPTER ONE

The Simplified Guide to Understanding Brain Training

The brain, in actuality, it is effectively the most entangled gadget on the planet. The craft of understanding in comprehensively having been an accomplishment endeavored to many, however, accomplished by none so far. Notwithstanding leaps forward in innovation have allowed specialists the methods for heightening their understanding of it to the following dimension. One of the surprising outcomes from this is brain training; exactly planned exercises that are equipped for improving your intellectual capacity, focus, creativity, memory, and even in scholastics. This guide will give you a short prologue to brain training and the components that make it so useful.

Tactile Manipulation

We all know that we have all the five detects that are our site, contact, taste, smell, and hearing. These five components are various roads for information to be moved to our brain before it's processed into recollections and encounters. This incorporates the smallest things, similar to how warmth feels, or even how your companion resembles. Backing out this information moving the process is as necessary as having the option to recollect more subtleties to keep your brain from filling the questions with spaces and resulting in disarray, wrong observations, and impediments. The brain training abuses this process by improving your physical capacities. The activity is focused on expanding the general edge of putting away information and enhances the quality that accompanies it by recollecting unpretentious subtleties. This additionally triggers a ripple effect, improving increasingly muddled elements of the brain.

Brain Degeneration

As we become more seasoned, our brains deny in terms of processing time, strength, and exactness. This converts into entirely detectable contrasts as you age. The brain training understands this inadequacy, yet the ideal approach to move you around it is to begin as ahead of schedule as could be expected under the circumstances. During the ages of youth, the brain is the most undeveloped, practically equal to be a plant that has not been watered. The brain training is the fundamental supplements that the plant requires. Generally, its development won't be amplified, and its potential won't be completely figured it out. This requires a more prominent requirement for brain training in children also because their prime age enables them to be increasingly retentive to the exercises, resulting in quickened results. These two components of the brain training are the minimum necessities of brain training and convert into the accompanying articulation. The brain training is best in children, and it is entirely workable for them to develop in terms of certainty, creativity, memory, and character development.

This Is The Most Powerful Tool To Maximize Brain Function
Exercise is the single most potent apparatus we have to maximize our brain function. This is because of the extensive cascade of chemical compounds, including hormones, neurotransmitters, and growth factors, that are unleashed in and into the brain when we get in a decent exercise. A bit of history to explain how we realize this is in order. In the late twentieth century, scientists discovered an ordinarily occurring compound in the brain and named it Brain-Derived Neurotrophic Factor, or BDNF. They found that when brain cells resting comfortably in a petri dish were sprinkled with BDNF, they started growing - sprouting dendrites like distraught - similar to what they do as a component of our brain's mass when we are learning something new. Since then, there have been a considerable number of research papers written about BDNF. In these multiple studies, researchers have found that when this compound is activated, it acts to protect brain cells from deterioration, strengthens neural connections, and even stimulates the birth of new brain cells. Close on the heels of this ground-breaking research, Carl Cotman at the University of California, Irvine's Institute for Brain Aging and Dementia was studying why some older people remain mentally sharp the entirety of their days while others suffer severe cognitive decline. He found that those who keep their mental faculties completely functioning as they age shared three characteristics practically speaking: education, and exercise. Wondering why physical

exercise would improve and maintain one's mental clarity, he devised an experiment to see if yoga would increase the release of BDNF in the brain. Since few individuals wish to donate their brains to research while they are still using them, he enlisted the help of some very enthusiastic mice. Correctly, Cotman put a running wheel in the cages of some of the rodent "volunteers." The mice were divided into gatherings that approached an operating motor two days, four days, or seven days a week, or not in the slightest degree. He found that the mice loved to run in the wheel to the tune of several kilometers (a few miles) per night. When Cotman later dissected the brains of the now-less-than-enthusiastic mice, he found that the exercise had significantly increased the measure of BDNF in the brain. That, however, the more the fuzzy little volunteers had run (e.g., four days versus two days), the more of this brain-cell-growing substance had been produced AND it was found in substantial sums in the hippocampus - the region of the brain primarily responsible for learning and memory! BDNF, however, is merely one of the compounds that flood the brain when we burn some calories. With each exercise, IGF-1 (insulin-like growth factor) is released from storage in the liver and other pieces of the body to help with metabolizing glucose to produce energy and after that travels by bloodstream through the blood-brain barrier into the brain where it changes roles to improve to learn. Additionally released with exercise and subsequently entering the brain is FGF-2 (fibroblast growth factor). Once in the brain, FGF-2 is instrumental in turning the hippocampus' stem cells into mature brain cells, a process called neurogenesis (i.e., the creation of new brain cells). Be that as it may, that is not all by far. Exercise signals the release of a multitude of chemical compounds that improve our state of mind, dull pain, keep us motivated and attentive and generally help our cognition. Here are a few of these compounds:

1. Anandamide and Endocannabinoids - These compounds connect to the same receptor sites that marijuana's THC uses, improving the state of mind and pleasure.

2. Dopamine - One of the brain's neurotransmitters, it has to do with maintaining attention, staying motivated, and

feelings of pleasure.

3. Serotonin - This neurotransmitter helps quell anxiety and impulsivity.

4. ANP (atrial natriuretic peptide) - ANP is a substance produced in the heart when the heart beats faster; it travels to the brain where it assumes a role in calming feelings of stress and anxiety.

5. VEGF ((vascular endothelial growth factor) - This compound helps create new blood vessels (capillaries) to help and supply newly formed brain cells.

That is only some of the cascade of chemicals that is set into motion when we get ourselves into action. Incidentally, those new brain cells that are created in the hippocampus when we exercise, they have only 28 days to get their demonstration together, or they get "washed away." In other words, the exercise gets the brain cells ready to learn, however then we have to learn something or explore new territory and different, or we lose the newly formed neurons. To keep our brain growing, therefore, we need to take dancing lessons, learn a foreign language, solve a puzzle, prepare a new recipe, drive a new route home or ________.
Presently you know! The most potent instrument for optimal brain function is heart-thumping, muscular contracting exercise followed by learning something new or doing something that challenges the mind! What are you going to do with this knowledge?

How to Renew an Aging Brain
We realize that care of the brain is fundamental for the stupendous children. Shouldn't something be said about us- - the nearly or more than sixty-somethings? What goes for the little ones goes for us too!
My mom used to state that her brain was stuck in concrete. She would never learn as fast as we (the kids) did because her brain had solidified with age. This suspicion about the brain has been hurled aside as another urban legend down the residue. New research shows that neuroplasticity is an element all things considered, youthful and old. This means whether you are 90 or 2,

you are capable of learning new traps.

Neuroplasticity alludes to the brain's ability to adjust to its condition. It can produce new neuronal hardware, new cells, make up for shortcoming by supplanting malfunctioning connections and cells with new ones. Nothing in the brain is designed. Like the lizard that can recover its tail, the brain can re-develop new neurons. It is this repaying instrument that indicates the way brain longevity. We need not relegate ourselves to the destiny of moderate and palsied years. Aging isn't synonymous with the loss of memory and individual abilities. What would we be able to do to guarantee a flourishing brain in our senior years?

Break Out Of Routine

Researchers have discovered that visual deficiency from birth can trigger the advancement of a visual cortex that can hear and feel. The brain area gave to sight has been recruited by the auditory function. Individuals dazzle since birth are truly capable of understanding with their eyes or looking with their ears. We can improve our multi-adroitness by accomplishing something extraordinary: take another course to work, travel to another nation, learn another language, and learn another aptitude. Accomplishing something strange powers your brain to cut new courses, increase synaptic connections, and supersede out of date circuits.

Begin Running

Ongoing studies on aerobic action and brain function have turned out some intriguing actualities: aerobic preparing increases brain volume in more seasoned grown-ups while non-aerobic activities, for example, extending and conditioning don't create a similar impact; seniors who are aerobically prepared appear to be increasingly capable of continued attention; they are less susceptible to diversions. Tests likewise uncover that seniors engaged in aerobic preparing scored fundamentally preferred on neuropsychological tests over their non-aerobic colleagues. Cardio workouts, like running, appear to disintegrate the impacts of negative weight on the brain and support the body's safe framework.

Develop a Passion

Faced with a challenging situation, our brains are compelled to grow new systems and new neural circuits. In any case, faced with a challenging job that we cherish, that positively energizes us, our brains are influenced to manufacture new neural discussions between various pieces of the brain. Passion gives the lubricating catalyst to increased synaptic terminating and connections, a situation promoted by the adage, "Cells that fire together stay wired together." This is the reason we learn quite a lot more quickly when we are energized by the material we work with, be it another leisure activity, a book taking shape or another business. if, as studies propose, aging is brought about by a dramatic decrease in functional connections inside the brain, at that point developing a passion is a sure-fire way to fire up a disturbed framework.

Meditate

Centered attention during meditation modifies the structure of the brain. Studies show that regular meditators enact the prefrontal cortex that is situated at the front of the brain; in the meantime, the limbic segment of the brain located at the back backs off. It is this attention that advances neuroplasticity in the brain. Besides, meditation increases the thickness of the cortex, the outside area of the brain most susceptible to age-related diminishing. This increase in thickness is regularly connected with the ability to incorporate feelings and thought the left brain and the right brain. The issue with healthy aging isn't so much skin revived with Botox or liposuction of fat tissues, yet a solid and subjectively sharp brain. This we can have available to us without an enormous cost. All we have to do are four things: break out of routine, go for a run, support a passion and meditate.

Your Brain Needs Three Things

Before we talk about the three things, your brain needs, we should take a gander at how seriously your brain needs them and that they are so crucial to your survival.

Your brain weighs just around 3 pounds, which speaks to about 2% of your total body weight. Incredibly, however, it devours 25% of the glucose that your body converts and 25% of the oxygen you take in. Does that appear somewhat uneven perhaps narrow-minded to you? It does to me at first look however the fact of the matter is your brain gains all of the vitality it detracts from the rest of the body. Imaging running up a trip of stairs; except if you are a prepared competitor, you will rapidly come up short on oxygen and start to gasp. When gasping isn't sufficient to keep you running, you need to stop and recoup let the lungs get. Consider the possibility that what happened to the brain. You think and think and concentrate until your brain can't keep up and you need to stop. Your brain runs each other piece of the body; not exclusively might you be able not to figure, your heart would stop siphoning, your lungs stop breathing, your eyes stop seeing, your ears stop hearing and your skeletal - solid framework stop working and you would crumble. If you had been pondering how to make tracks in the opposite direction from moving toward tyrannosaurs, you would be in absolute chaos. So honors to our brains for having the option to work 24x7, performing various tasks billions of subtleties and organizing our creatures for quite a long time. Presently the issue turns out to be how long? Science is in understanding that our brainpower peaks in the mid-twenties at that point begins to decline. Research likewise demonstrates that at age 55, our brain power has been decreased by half of what it was in the mid-twenties. The decline proceeds and quickens, and when we are eighty, 33% of us have been determined to have some dementia, similar to Alzheimer's or AAMI. At age 85 the percentage increases to half. Since therapeutic science is giving us a chance to live, brain decline is ending up increasingly predominant and all the more an issue. We need to begin focusing on the brain with what it needs to remain essential and useful our whole lives not simply until retirement. So what does your brain require to stay in the game? Help it is essential for your brain to slow down and rest. Cortisol is a synthetic your body produces when under stress; it is dangerous to the brain. When you don't give the brain a chance to escape from the pressure cooker on a customary basis, the stress hormone builds up, and the neurons and synapses separate. The brain will make up for the damaged purchase plunging into stores yet without a dipstick to quantify what's left your brain can and will come up short. You would feel that rest, and resting the brain explicitly would be simple; however, it requires exertion.

Exercise-use it or free it. Research has demonstrated that the more you invigorate and think carefully, the better it progresses toward becoming and the more it keeps going. Recreations and riddles that make you believe are great; however, don't give them a chance to wind up routine, or you will invalidate the point. Inventive undertakings like stitching or building perch rooms drive you to think. Learning to play a melodic instrument; learning to move or fly fish are excellent. Things that are new and distinctive driving you to think and figure things out will fabricate and save your brain for quite a long time.

Nutrition-the brain needs nutrition, and it is ending up increasingly evident every year that what we feed the brain needs to be explicit brain nutrition. Fish truly is brain food, so are broccoli and Brussels grows, nuts and beans; not your regular Mickey Ds lunch reasonable. It truly is challenging to eat everything you have to keep up mental and physical wellbeing. Regardless of whether you begin today on a brain explicit eating routine will your body ever have the option to process enough nutrition to keep up your brain not to mention restore it?

CHAPTER TWO

Yoga For Your Brain

It has been examined and demonstrated that yoga meditation practices positively affect animating your brain. Yoga, meditation, and deep breathing are known to decrease anxiety and stress. Another positive symptom is improved focus when taking part in various undertakings.

The Mayo Clinic and the University of California, L.A., just as other research gatherings, have discovered that by rehearsing yoga for as meager as 12 minutes per day reliably for a multi-month time frame, helps to decrease stress levels and anxiety. We realize that stress can lead to numerous health issues as it makes our resistant framework become kindled. This inflammation leaves us progressively helpless against different health issues, one being misery.

Yoga and meditation instruct you to focus on your breath. This focus is accepted to increase brain function and memory. It additionally helps to keep you in the present as opposed to being engrossed with what's to come. This necessary demonstration of living in the present is known to increase our general joy.

Yoga and controlled breathing trigger biochemical changes in our brain. It helps secure our telomeres, which leads to lower rates of infection. "A telomere is an area of redundant DNA toward the end of a chromosome, which shields the end of the chromosome from decay." (News Medical)

Yoga has been connected with boosting your GABA levels. It invigorates a piece of your sensory system, which appears to lead you to a condition of quiet. Quiet leads to better dispositions and more vitality. We, as a whole, realize that stress is depleting both rationally and physically.

So snatch your yoga mat and attempt some stress alleviation presents. The following are some high stances for stress and anxiety.

- Sukhasana (Easy Pose)

- Marjaryasana (Cat Pose)
- Bitilasana (Cow Pose)
- Balasana (Child's Pose)
- Uttana Shishosana (Extended Puppy Pose)
- Adho Mukha Svanasana (Downward Facing Dog)
- Setubandhasana (Bridge Pose)
- Uttanasana (Standing Forward Bend)
- Paschimottanasana (Seated Forward Bend)
- Salamba Sirasana (Supported Headstand)

It is ideal to end your practice with Savasana (Corpse Pose). It's an excellent method to calm your body alongside your mind. Rests on your yoga mat on your in an agreeable and common position with your palms looking up. You should remain in this situation for at any rate of five minutes. Before rising, take a couple of profound breathes in and breathes out. At that point gradually roll onto your right side and utilize your arms and hands to sit progressively up, raising your head last.

Continuously wipe down your yoga mat after each practice to keep it spotless and new.

Namaste.

Yoga is an excellent method to de-stress through extending and meditation. It helps improve focus, which continues to your regular exercises. All you need is a tranquil spot and an agreeable yoga mat. Appreciate yoga for your healthy - mind and body.

Super Brain Yoga

Super Brain Yoga is the most effortless, quickest, and least complicated form of exercise that is internationally practiced today for energizing and adjusting the brain. It is one of the comprehensive approaches to revive and strengthen, particularly after pressure and mind numbering action. This form of yoga is principally founded on simple techniques of acupuncturing your ears. The practitioners need to hold their tongue up to the top of their mouth to finish the course of energy Meridians. This technique opens the Eustachian tubes accessible in your ears through which energy streams in. It is the quickest form of exercise where you don't need to spend extended periods rehearsing it..

Logically approved technique, Super Brain Yoga is universally acclaimed for energizing the brain of the practitioners and even improves clarity and sharpness. Grand Master Choa Kok Sui has created this straightforward and quickest technique with an expectation to improve the scholarly limit of individuals and to sharpen both concentration and memory. The original focal point of this form of exercise is to enable energy to spill out of the lower power focuses or lower chakras to the crown chakras and temple. In this procedure, the heat is consequently changed into inconspicuous energy, and thus, it is utilized by your brain to improve its functioning and concentration.

Instructions to Practice

It is said that this form of yoga ought to be practiced early toward the beginning of the day to appreciate most extreme advantages from it. It tends to be practiced anyplace in the home. However, it would be better if it is performed amidst some peaceful and serene environs. Expel your ear gems before starting this exercise and hold your right ear with the left hand, setting the thumb in the front side of the ear and remaining index finger in the posterior of the ear. Also, hold the left ear with your right hand in the same style. Keep in mind, when you sit holding your ear, you need to breathe in profoundly while returning to standing position you need to breathe out bit by bit.

Advantages of Super Brain Yoga

- It enacts and empowers your brain.
- It improves your internal peace
- It decreases mental pressure and even offers your extraordinary mental stability
- Enhances your knowledge and creativity
- Regulates sex drive
- Partial energizing and cleansing effects on emanations and chakras
- Conversion of lower energies into higher energies
- Increasing the functioning of the brain

- Regular rehearsing of this exercise will make the practitioners more astute and mental adjusted
- Spiritual development

Significant Points

- While performing this exercise, you need to wear free outfits and attempt to spruce up with agreeable pieces of clothing to complete this workout serenely.
- Pregnant ladies are encouraged to counsel their social insurance supplier before starting with this workout regime.
- The best time to practice this form of exercise is early morning hour or late at night.
- Effective outcomes can be accomplished if it is practiced with void stomach
- Ensure that you usually exercise and bit by bit to appreciate exceptional outcomes from it.

Yoga Psychology

One of the more delightfully created sciences of spiritual-based psychology is yoga psychology, the study of the human psyche in connection to life and the more significant components of existence. This science, registered from the old convention of yoga, seeks to clarify and investigate the possibilities of the human life, revealing the shrouded riddles behind life's motivation, existence, and relationship to the world in which we live. While there are numerous systems of psychology accessible to current man, yoga psychology is one of a kind in that is seeks to consolidate present-day science with antiquated philosophy. Through its particular methods of treating and transforming the mind to its open and all-encompassing way to deal with life, yoga psychology is a viable science for giving a healthy, adjusted, and individually delicate methodology the psychological wellness and wellbeing.

The Philosophy of Psychology

Generally, the philosophy of psychology has sought after two outlets. The primary recommends that life is empirical and can be estimated and observed on a physical level. This philosophy keeps up that all system is composed of the issue which can be seen through physical perception and followed through the faculties. In this way, everything that exists inside the human being can be estimated on a physical level accounts for all aspects of human existence. A critical purpose of this philosophical belief system is that everything is dependent on experience, outside info, and hereditary aura. These together form the whole establishment for the psyche. Along these lines, elements that seem to reach out past the limits of the physical and noticeable level of existence are either envisioned or yet to be proven through empirical perception.

In opposition to the empirical belief is the philosophy that human beings are composed of elements that are past the bounds of the physical structure of the human being. Albeit material components add to our existence, numerous features of the human nature can't be estimated with a magnifying lens or electromagnetic outputs although these features are not composed of a similar material as the human body, their existence in their measurement and hold the characteristics that enable them to exist. One of the essential instances of an element that exists in its form is consciousness. Under the meaning of the non-empirical philosophy, knowledge is a part of human life, however, isn't contained exclusively inside the human being, nor would it be able to be found inside the structures of the brain. Or maybe it is a field of existence that saturates all of creation, however, takes the presence of isolated substances when separated through the structure of the individual elements, for example, a human being. In this manner, it is part of the human being, yet not constrained to the human structure all by itself. Generally, empirical based psychology accepts that consciousness is a component of the brain, and a spirit, or some entity that is associated with a higher source, does not exist. All that is experienced and seen inside the individual can be clarified inside the physical substance of the human being. In this way, the quest for understanding and appreciation of the functions of the human psyche are, for the most part, attempted inside the study of the brain through the sciences, for example, neuropsychology. This forms the establishment for the more expanded investigations of conduct, formative, and intellectual psychology. Non-empirical psychology, then again, acknowledges the spirit, or something existing with the human being that stretches out past the breaking points of the transitory body, as the other entity adding to the human existence. While the human body contains part of the material essential to form life, it doesn't make up the entire system. Nonexperimental psychology keeps up the belief that individual consciousness is a component of an extensive system that has been alluded to as vast, widespread, or aggregate consciousness. In light of this understanding, non-empirical psychology seeks after the study of the human psyche through the components of consciousness, soul/spirit, and different elements past the physical body. While few out of every odd psychology conforms to these limits, the majority of the applied practices of psychology conform themselves to the diagram of one of this belief system; either the mind is in the body and the brain, or it is part of something bigger and past the cutoff points of the body. As a social practice, western psychology, as a rule, pursues the way of the empirical study, whereas eastern psychology has been that of the metaphysical and spiritualistic. However, there are present-day ways of thinking, scientists, and therapists that are reaching out past these limits and looking to reform psychology into a total science of the human mind. Undoubtedly, the human brain shows outstanding commitments to the functions of an idea, observation, and conduct, and yet there has been no significant proof that mindfulness or consciousness can be contained inside the features of the brain. Together, both of these bits of knowledge have proven to be considerable difficulties to the cutting edge research of the psychology of human beings. Yoga Psychology, as a traditional practice, has advanced to embody both the empirical and non-empirical point of view of psychology. In spite of the fact that it could generally be considered a non-empirical philosophy, yoga psychology has likewise extraordinarily acknowledged the impacts of the anatomical structure in creating, molding, and making the psychology of a human being; yet the physical body does not contain the majority of the elements essential to form the multifaceted nature of the human mind and consciousness. Through the philosophy and spiritual-probe of yoga, yoga psychology keeps up the belief that the human psychology is formed by variables from the different circle of life, beginning from the most material physical body and working through to the unobtrusive elements of the spirit. Each layer isn't a free system, nor is it contained inside one single structure. Or maybe, there are a few sheaths that exist together and work flawlessly between each other to form the entire structure, form, and existence of the human being.

The Application of Psychology

Psychology is intended to be applied as a practical way to provide people with a healthy mind. While the meaning of what establishes a healthy mind may fluctuate between various philosophical beliefs, generally people need carry on with a life that contains more bliss, a more grounded self-idea, and a character that is equipped for dealing with the changes and advancing occasions in life. Psychology seeks to provide people with the apparatuses essential to make the right conditions for a healthy mind, utilizing an assortment of aptitudes, observations, and methods to help form the ideal outcomes. Among a portion of the real components used by modern psychology to help people locate a healthier mental develop include: medication, counseling, bunch treatment, psycho-examination, genetic modifications, and spiritual molding. These methods look to provide people with a more grounded mental state with which they can approach life. "Normal" forms of psychology, for the most part, maintain a strategic distance from medication and shifty techniques that may make further changes to the bio-compound structure of the body. They additionally customarily center around moving toward psychological edifices with a progressively all-encompassing point of view which incorporates physical infirmities and enthusiastic disturbances. Conversely, a more "westernized" system of psychology, as a rule, treats patients dependent on ordered issue or dysfunctions which are identified with the mind or the brain. Treatment is provided dependent on the side effects of a patient about other traditionally characterized cases. For some patients, medication is utilized related to counseling and therapy. As a practice, yoga psychology, for the most part, tends to the psychological changes inside a human being's life with a wide assortment of techniques, each intended to help direct and adjust a particular inconsistency inside the human system. Generally, yoga psychology pursues the "characteristic" policy of mental healthcare as it ordinarily treats each case freely, assisting an individual after investigation of the physical, psychological, lively, and spiritual elements of their life. For physical disturbances, which are influencing the mental state, exercise, and development known as the asanas (stances) are applied. These can likewise be utilized related to purging techniques which help to expel poisons from the body. For psychological disturbances, contemplation, fixation, and self-perception are being used. Generally, the body and the mind are seen as reliant elements, so precise physical movement or changes can regard psychological disturbances too. For vital issues, breathing activities are utilized to increment or lessening vitality inside the body. Diet can likewise be changed to help increment essentialness. The health of the spiritual aspect of life is reliant on the state of the physical, mental, and enthusiastic bodies, and in this manner is commonly thought about by treating these bodies first.

Albeit numerous systems of psychology exist, yoga psychology is one that can be applied for the individuals who look for superior information of themselves. While a belief in spiritual aspects of life will help one who wishes to practice yoga psychology, it's anything but a need. Or maybe, yoga psychology ought to be seen as an all-encompassing system of psychology which works to make a harmony in the body and the mind with the goal that ideal health and quality can be accomplished. It likewise works to provide people with a more prominent understanding of life as the body, mind, and spirit are effectively transformed to achieve their fullest possibilities.

Yoga For Intelligence
There is an assortment of Yoga techniques that enhance intelligence and help one settle on intelligent decisions. Yoga techniques that improve the subjective working of the brain incorporate inversion asanas that increase the course of fresh recruits and oxygen into the brain. Yoga pranayama techniques that help to subdue nervousness, likewise support a Yoga expert in precisely getting to a situation, without the perplexity of a restless,

dashing, and overactive personality. Moreover, Yoga asanas and reflection techniques, which request a one-pointed focus, help a Yogi or Yogini to focus on one task at a time. This ability to focus supports an astute evaluation of a situation and enhances the professional's ability to finish on one job at a time in everyday life. The accompanying inversion poses will flip around your reality! Both of these Yoga asanas help to flow fresh blood and oxygen all through the body, including the brain. With an increase of fresh blood and oxygen, the brain will work all the more effectively, and brain fogginess will be mitigated - in this way, improving intelligence.

Legs up the Wall - Viparita Karani
To rehearse Legs up the Wall pose, place your Yoga mat in a wrong position. Hurry your sit bones sideways against the wall, and after that slowly raise your legs the wall, in an opposite view, to the floor. This pose is extremely therapeutic, and you will get a considerable lot of similar advantages of Shoulder Stand or Head Stand, without taking a considerable risk. Remain in this pose for up to five or ten minutes, and after that descend slowly, resting for a couple of minutes in a fetal position.

Supported Shoulder Stand - Salamba Sarvangasana
Shoulder stand is a more profound and more extreme inversion. Soak inversions are enabling. Be that as it may, individuals with prior neck issues, high or low blood weight, a past stroke, heart issues, epilepsy, confined retina, or glaucoma ought to counsel their doctor or expert before endeavoring them. To practice Shoulder Stand, place a folded blanket on your Yoga mat at shoulder tallness. Rests on the coverage and ensure that your shoulders meet the edge of the folded blanket, however don't hang over the edge. Slowly, raise your legs not yet decided and opposite to the floor. Support your torso with your hands at your lower back. Keep your arms tucked perfectly into your sides. Broaden your legs further up towards the ceiling. Hold Shoulder Stand for three to five minutes, or anyway long feels suitable for you today. When you are prepared to descend, bring down your legs slowly withdraw to the floor, as you take off of the pose, vertebrae by vertebrae. Kindly do Fish Pose as a counter-pose in

the wake of rehearsing Shoulder Stand. Fish Pose is performed by setting your hands, palms down, under your sacrum territory, elbows tucked perfectly into your sides, as you curve your torso up towards the ceiling, while you open your neck and throat region to the sky. Descend slowly and rest in Corpse Pose.

Both of these inversion stances will enhance intelligence, by coursing fresh recruits and crisp oxygen all through the whole body, including the brain. Pranayama Yoga techniques and other Yoga asanas, that lower uneasiness levels and require extraordinary fixation and focus, will likewise enhance intelligence.

The Human Mind and Yoga

These days it is essential to have a peaceful mind. The vast majority of the complexities or sicknesses that the body may experience are the aftereffect of a grieved soul. As indicated by a psychologist, the brain can be affected by a few external variables, and these components can add to the conduct of a person paying little respect to its effect. By and large, a person who is experiencing an excessive amount of stress is portrayed with bothersome manner. Psychologists accept that fear can hinder and reduce the normal behavior of a person since it, for the most part, focuses on the mind. The brain is considered as the control system of the entire human body. The one coordinates messages and motivations all through the body. Anyway, the brain is just the physical or physiological part of the control system. The one that performs the obligation or assignment of controlling the entire human body is the mind. The mind is the person who examines the things that wander around the system of the body. It is additionally the one which is dependable in making any forms of reactions towards nature or the extreme condition. Since the mind is necessary, we should take the most secure approach to maintain its equalization and sound condition. Guarding the account against any forms of threat is a perfect yet a troublesome errand to maintain. It requires the consideration and readiness of a person. The mind must be treated as a standout amongst the most precious adornments since it is without a doubt so. There are a few hints on how you can dispose of environmental stress that imperils the mindset of a person. As indicated by a psychologist, a strategy with no forms of drugs or prescription is the ideal approach to get a calm and sound mind. It must be all characteristic and natural. It is because any kinds of drugs or meds can influence the general state of the brain. Yoga has been a standout amongst the best strategies that are being drilled by Hindus. The activity portrays their way of life and convictions. The people who take part in this specific kind of training are called Yogi. The standards of yoga are genuinely philosophical since it incorporates their beliefs about oneself and the proliferation of the mind. During the introduction of yoga, individuals are utilizing it to look for the information of knowing themselves. It expects to bind together nature and the spirit of human creatures. Yoga frequently incorporates physical activity. Extending is the first advance in performing this sort of activity. It is essential to utilize the best possible kinds of equipment with regards to this activity since it is inclined to mishaps. Appropriate yoga clothing is likewise required for the individuals who need to rehearse yoga since it enables its members to extend their bodies without stressing over their appearance. Yoga clothing and equipment can be purchased in a few yoga clothing stores. It is essential to buy from an affirmed yoga clothing store to keep you from purchasing counterfeit things that are generally unsatisfactory.

The Many Benefits of Yoga and Fitness
Many people are attempting to improve their health nowadays, and regularly, people look to new ways in which to do this. Dieting is a craze of the past, and even traditional exercise is being pushed aside for new techniques that guarantee to burn fat and tone muscles. Yoga is one of those new ways to get your body fit as a fiddle. Not to say that a healthy diet isn't necessary; however, matched with regular yoga workouts, you will be amazed at the results. What's more, yoga isn't just for physical health either; the benefits go well past the physical aspect.
Since the physical benefits that you get from yoga are so significant, we will talk about them first. Yoga makes it workable for us to train our bodies to use correct posture regardless of what we are doing. The various poses help to tone the muscles in our body as well as train them too. Yoga likewise works to improve blood flow through breathing techniques, which assists body gain the measure of oxygen essential. The majority of this causes the

cerebrum to function correctly. Although these may not be aspects of physical health that we frequently consider, improving such issues will surely provide a distinction in the way that we feel. The second most important benefit that you will gain from practicing yoga has to do with the mind. Yoga is an incredible way to loosen up the mind and reduce stress brought on by everyday life. The techniques practiced, including the postures just as the breathing is intended to sooth the mind and soul and enable us to relinquish negative energy. Practicing yoga additionally will assist you with connecting your mind and body better too. This by itself can significantly reduce stress in both the body and mind, which gives us an over generally improved feeling. Yoga has many health benefits too. The decrease of stress and the physical improvements combine to provide us with over altogether improved health by and large. A healthy body and mind result in a healthy immune system which will assist you with fighting off sickness and disease. Practicing yoga will likewise enable you to keep up a healthy weight, increment your physical energy, improve your memory and readiness, and even keep your body feeling good regardless of physical exertion. The general feeling of wellbeing will be a standard part of your life not long after you start practicing yoga techniques. Choosing to assume control over your life and focusing on any routine is a significant decision. Before starting any diet or any exercise routine individuals ought to counsel their doctor. Yoga is a relatively safe practice, yet those that have balance issues may need to discover ways to help themselves to ensure their physical safety. Before starting, you may likewise need to buy a comfortable mat to use during your routine, and you will need to locate a comfortable place to work out in too. A little while later, you will start to feel the many benefits of practicing yoga and will before long feel superior to ever. Many people are attempting to improve their health nowadays, and regularly, people look to new ways in which to do this. Dieting is a trend of the past, and even traditional exercise is being pushed aside for new techniques that guarantee to burn fat and tone muscles. Yoga is one of those new ways to get your body fit as a fiddle. Not to say that a healthy diet isn't vital; however, matched with regular yoga workouts, you will be astonished at the results. Also, yoga isn't just for physical health either. The benefits go well past the physical aspect. Since the physical benefits that you get from yoga are so significant, we will talk about them first. Yoga makes it feasible for us to train our bodies to use correct posture regardless of what we are doing. The various stances help to tone the muscles in our body as well as train them also. Yoga likewise works to improve blood flow through breathing techniques, which assists body gain the measure of oxygen essential. The majority of this encourages the cerebrum to function correctly. Although these may not be aspects of physical health that we regularly consider, improving such issues will surely provide a distinction in the way that we feel. The second most important benefit that you will gain from practicing yoga has to do with the mind. Yoga is an extraordinary way to loosen up the mind and reduce stress brought on by everyday life. The techniques practiced, including the stances just as the breathing is intended to sooth the mind and soul and enable us to relinquish negative energy. Practicing yoga likewise will assist you with connecting your mind and body better too. This by itself can significantly reduce stress in both the body and mind, which gives us an over generally improved feeling.

Yoga has many health benefits too. The decrease of stress and the physical improvements combine to provide us with over altogether improved health when all is said in done. A healthy body and mind result in a healthy immune system which will assist you with fighting off illness and disease. Practicing yoga will likewise enable you to keep up a healthy weight, increment your physical energy, improve your memory and readiness, and even keep your body feeling good regardless of physical exertion. The general feeling of health will be a standard part of your life not long after you start practicing yoga techniques. Choosing to assume control over your life and focusing on any routine is a significant decision. Before starting any diet or any exercise routine individuals ought to counsel their doctor. Yoga is a relatively safe practice; however, those that have balance issues may need to discover ways to help themselves to ensure their physical safety. Before starting, you may likewise need to buy a comfortable mat to use during your routine, and you will need to locate a comfortable place to work out in also. After a short time, you will start to feel the many benefits of practicing yoga and will before long feel over anyone's imagination.

CHAPTER THREE
Exercise - Tying it All Together

I complete a lot of writing and speaking regarding the matter of exercise and fitness, particularly cardiovascular and resistance training. I talk about the importance of incorporating intensity and variety into our exercise, doing full body resistance training, mixing up cardio training with low burst-like activity just as perseverance like activity (if you appreciate it), at the same time remembering to include your flexibility, posture, and proprioceptive exercise.

Hold up! Sounds like a lot.
As a result, I'm regularly asked, "How would you fit it all in?"
"Any way I can!" is the legitimate answer! I don't have one precisely perfect way for that I approach fitting in the various types of exercise. There IS nobody precisely the ideal way! The most critical piece of this entire exercise and time management puzzle is to decide that you WILL fit it in, regardless. That has been the most crucial factor for me. Sometimes, plans change, or there's a severe conflict of my schedule, and I'm not ready to stick to my original exercise plan for the afternoon. Having decided that I will move my body daily enables me to quickly shift apparatuses and accomplish something else to meet my body's innate genetic requirements for exercise — not a major ordeal. Move! Alright, so past deciding to exercise and move forever, I've separated my exercise regime into four main components: resistance training, cardiovascular exercise, posture and proprioception, and flexibility/yoga. There's some cover in this component - don't sweat the details!

Resistance Training:
I believe, and research confirms, that high intensity, varied full body resistance training is the superior strategy for working out. This is the number one way to build slender muscle which, in turn, most effectively consumes fat and calories. My resistance training workouts are typically 25-45 minutes long. They are quick-paced, concentrated sessions that emphasis on big, multi-joint, functional

exercises in request to make the highest workload for my body, and in this manner, the best results. Depending on my disposition and what other workouts I've been doing, 2/3 of the time, I'll include "power" to these workouts. I'll consist of burst-like moves, like squat bounces, vertical jumps, seat hops, and so forth. I generally do these workouts three times every week. I include abdominal exercises toward the finish of these sessions. I work out at home, so I don't have any childcare issues to manage. I'd want to do these workouts in the morning to maximize the metabolic impacts of resistance training, yet our exercise room is right by where the kids rest... it is highly unlikely I'm going to wake the sleeping bears! I do resistance training in the midday after work, and homeschooling items have been tended to. The kids realize I'm going to fit my workouts in a few times every week. They're frequently in the life with me, joining in or doing their very own thing. It's a piece of their life, as well.

Cardiovascular Exercise:
I would get outside and go for a long run or bike ride each day if my schedule permitted... also if it were the best thing for my body. My plan doesn't take into consideration that kind of time daily, and that sort of exercise isn't ideal daily at any rate. Again, science shows that high intensity, widely varied exercise is ideal. This implies it benefits us to mix things up. My cardio is a mix of longer runs and bike rides (an hour or progressively), short, burst-like runs and sprinting sessions... what's more, combinations of the two. More than once every week, I want to get out for a longer run. In any event one time for every week, my cardio exercise is centered around short, intense bursts — for instance, a 20-minute session of hill sprints. Different times, I'll mix it up a bit: a middle distance run with specific races or quicker running on the uphills. Since I have the kids at home throughout the day, and they're too youthful to be in any way taken off alone, my significant other and I alternate fitting in our cardio workouts. I wait until he gets back home at lunch to go out on some weekdays, in addition to I'll provide in several sessions on the weekend. At that point, there are all the different cardio sessions, like running here and there hills with the kids on one of our "tendency stroll," and jumping on the trampoline, and pulling the kids in the trailer behind the bike,

etc. Those are merely icing on the cake! With everything taken into account, I typically do 'official' cardio exercise sessions 4-6 times for each week. Research exhibits that we needn't bother with this much cardio activity in request to achieve optimal Health and function. Be that as it may, each one of those smarty pants in research hasn't represented the amount I rationally and emotionally need this! Cardio is my number one pressure management device.

Posture and Proprioception (P&P):

When I first get up in the morning, way before the kids are done, I do about 10 or 15 minutes of specific movement and stretching to wake my body up and set it up for the afternoon, along with profound breathing exercises.

Since over half of proprioceptive input to the brain (the 'nourishment' that genuinely drives the brain's presentation) originates from the movement of the spine and its surrounding tissues, the majority of my proprioceptive exercises center around moving my entire needle. For instance, "Circles" exercise, just as cross-creep and twisting motions. The hips and lower legs are additionally great wellsprings of this neurological input for the brain, so I focus on those zones also. I additionally put in almost no time doing postural correction exercises. Anterior head carriage and rounding of the shoulders are very regular postural distortions that result in the absence of optimal function of the sensory system. Since I spend the first couple of hours of my day sitting at a PC, it's essential for me to counterbalance the negative postural impacts before I even begin. Finally, I do some hamstring, and hip flexor stretches toward the start of the day.

Flexibility/Yoga/Pilates:

This is the one class of exercise for me that covers with a portion of the others. I do some flexibility stretches in the mornings. However, I additionally do some when cardio and resistance. I might complete a yoga or Pilates floor routine on an 'off' day, or I might incorporate yoga postures and isometric training into a lighter resistance training day.

Despite how I fit it in, it's essential for me to fit it in! Resistance and cardio can get me up until this point. I think a big piece of expressing optimal Health and function throughout a lifetime is to be flexible just as powerful. I need to continue reminding myself to include this component... it's easier for me to get out and run than it is to back off and stretch!

With everything taken into account, some random week may resemble this:

Sunday - long distance run (or long bike ride)

Monday - start with P and P exercises and stretches.
- resistance training with "power."

Tuesday - start with P and P
- sprints

Wednesday - start with P and P
- resistance training with "power."

Thursday - start with P and P
- bright day, yoga, Pilates, walking, trampoline, and so forth.

Friday - start with P and P
- *long run*

Saturday - start with P and P
- Resistance training... what's more, perhaps a shorter, single run. Saturdays are generally the day for a family outing, like a long bike ride.
I typically interchange a cardio day with a resistance day. It's not frequently that I do cardio on a similar day as resistance training. If for reasons unknown I decide to, I do cardio following resistance training, and I won't include the "power" moves to the resistance session. Additionally, I'd be bound to complete one of the shorter, burst-like cardio sessions on a day when I combine the two kinds of exercise. Ideally, I do cardio and resistance on isolated days. Does my schedule always resemble this? Actually no, not ever. Sometimes, I jump on a move with running, and I'll complete a couple of days straight. Or then again, if I have an injury, I may

remove a day or two from the resistance training until my body repairs.

The details truly don't make a difference. What's important is to commit to giving your body what it needs - customary, varied movement. Motion is Life!

It is safe to say that you are bewildered by the overwhelming, regularly contradictory health information nowadays? Worried that your family may not be as healthy as they could be? So, you get a handle on focused and depleted... what's more, also darn tried to make positive, healthy lifestyle changes? I'm here to help! My name is Dr. Colleen Trombley, otherwise called Dr. Mother Online. I have a skill for simplifying Health and helping occupied ladies reestablish harmony to their lives. (Obviously, almost everything I educate likewise applies to men! Try not to stress, folks!)

The Powers of Meditation on the Anxious Brain

Meditation was always on my mind, yet for obvious reasons, I couldn't get to it. I was too caught up with being occupied, and with the measure of caffeine I was ingesting, I couldn't sit down and center around my musings, not notwithstanding for 2 minutes. Thus, quitting caffeine was central to my ability to meditate. A friend of mine suggested the book by Eckhart Tolle, The Power of Now, which laid down the foundation of meditation for me. It is an overwhelming book, and to be straightforward, I never finished it; however, what I read from it was sufficient to make me need to get familiar with it. During my research, I ran over the Integral Yoga Institute that offered a workshop called " Yoga-Based Cognitive-Behavioral Treatment of Anxiety" (when a month). The yoga instructor for this workshop is trained in psychotherapy, and as a result, the class was revolved around cognitive-behavioral treatment (CBT). There, I learned one type of meditation that energizes free-floating considerations. I was educated to relinquish any control and to watch and recognize whatever contemplations were coming through my mind. Indeed, it is that simple, however, just in principle, because in practice it is tough. The objective is to achieve a point where your mind all of a sudden turns out to be quiet, and all you see are lights and shapes.

I realize that since I have experienced it, and it is an excellent experience for somebody whose mind wouldn't stop. I did not achieve this state right away; it took a few sessions before I could finally experience the benefits of meditation for anxiety. I first started doing 5 minutes and after that moved on to 10 and 15 minutes. It was during the 15-minute session that I finally experienced a "clear mind," no musings, no images, just lights and moving shapes. It felt so great; I quickly wound up addicted to it.

The Power of Self-Awareness

The various types of meditation are each founded on a way of thinking, however they all objective an increase in mindfulness. Through meditation, one turns out to be increasingly attentive to one's considerations. Through meditation for anxiety, one turns out to be progressively mindful of one's anxious concerns. Mindfulness is a procedure by which we become mindful of our perspective, which in turn fortifies our feeling of self. Our lifestyle does not permit this kind of self-reflection since we don't have room schedule-wise to do as such. We may feel that it would be an exercise in futility since society has instilled in us the should be productive, and self-reflection does not fit the criteria. Mindfulness increases prosperity since considerations that were previously automatic and unconscious are currently raised to our attention. As a result, we have more command over them. That is the objective of Cognitive Behavioral Therapy (CBT). Clients are educated to monitor their upsetting musings to have the option to assess their rationality or their integrity, which in turn diminishes their grip over the individual. Sooner or later, the negative reflections become less and less overwhelming (see the previous post for more info o CBT). For my situation, through meditation, I had the option to identify and ruin those negative automatic considerations that exacerbated my anxiety, which at that point, enabled me to reduce my stress after some time.

A Quiet Mind

Another extraordinary benefit of meditation is the ability to experience quietness in mind. To explain this impact, I have to return to the idea of brain lateralization. In simple terms, the two cerebral cortices harbor distinct abilities (albeit not exclusively).

The left brain is logical and methodical. It thinks in language and procedure information linearly. The right brain, be that as it may, is mystical. It believes in pictures and procedure information as entire (vitality). Be that as it may, the vast majority of all, the left hemisphere is about the Past and the Future, while the Right region knows just the present minute. Meditation jolts the individual into the Present. It trains our brain to concentrate just on the present minute without any control or endeavor to change it. It is believed that meditation makes a parallel shift from left to right brain activity (although this hypothesis still requires further research). That is the point at which you achieve quietude. I experienced quietude after a few meditation sessions. It was tough because the brain babble (truly left brain prattle) would not stop. Indeed, it sensed that it was considerably more intense and all the more overwhelming while I was meditating; racing considerations, images being assaulted and even an obnoxious inner voice. Everything I could do was to give it a chance to occur, to make an effort not to control it, because, in the end, it would need to stop. As a similarity, it would be like letting a little child cry and shout while throwing an alter fit of rage until he quiets down individually. Along these lines, I let my mind meander indiscriminately without any constraints until one day a beautiful thing occurred. I had music in my mind. What was so beautiful about it was that I had not experienced music in a while, because the anxiety had hijacked my brain to the point of not being ready to hear music in my mind any longer. My brain was not playing melodies or even music pieces that I had heard previously and delighted in. It was all musings and jabber. In actuality, listening to music was insufferable because by one way or another, my brain couldn't filter it any longer, and as a result, it was unsavory and offensive. Along these lines, when I finally heard music in my mind, I started smiling since I had finally figured out how to quiet my left brain, and my right brain eventually dominated. I had made a colossal advance in the direction of controlling anxiety. I literally felt like I was spared. In additiln addition to music, I started visualizing lovely shapes (it is difficult to explain what was wonderful about them, they recently felt that way) and clear, bright lights, and that was the point at which the prattle would stop totally. No more sounds, it was as though somebody had squeezed the quiet catch on the remote control. For somebody living with anxiety, this silence is invaluable.

Modified Yoga Gives Relief for Depression and Anxiety
I have been teaching yoga for twenty-two years. I got into yoga at that time, since I was suicidal, not merely depressed. During that period, my state of mind, was down to the point that I started to fantasize always, on the most proficient method to kill myself. My friend hauled me to my first yoga class, and insisted, that yoga would help with my emotions. I resisted by saying, "By what method would yoga be able to help with your emotions?" I had done different exercises and different fitness classes. I was a sprinter, I played volleyball, basketball, tennis, and I did a wide range of fitness workouts. I dedicated myself entirely to weights, crunches, and sit-ups. I was tormented with stress, guilt, rage, insomnia, depression, and distress. Nothing had helped my state of mind until yoga. Yoga genuinely spared my life. Presently twenty after two years; I'm dedicated yoga teacher, with a passion for motivating, the individuals who are; depressed or suicidal; and I encourage them to come, to experience, the yoga difference. From the free first class that I tried, yoga was hard for me. The poses weren't that difficult to pursue, yet my hamstrings, hips, and back muscles were overly tight, and the stretching was painful for me. The breathing was in opposition to breathing in working out, where you inhale out, through your mouth, to maintain the power of the workout. In yoga, by comparison, you inhale continuously through your nose. You take full breaths in, that grow out your gut, and sometimes, you hold the inspiration for a few seconds. I was determined to figure yoga out. The developments were moderate and mindful. The repetitions of the event felt tedious. Yoga worked on your strength, and you needed to hold poses, for example, descending pooch, or board pose, or an inversion pose, for a few long moments. For what reason does modified yoga work to relieve depression and anxiety? I feel that it's a combination of elements. First, modified is a more comfortable yoga class than an ordinary beginner's course. I individual offer myself, and I urge clients to do precisely what each can do in my class. There is an acceptance, and spirituality that is present in a restorative or modified yoga class. The space in itself is very

calming and not intimidating. Yoga instructs you to stay in the present moment ultimately. To do the poses well, requires center, strength, balance, and a willingness to finish the pose. If your mind meanders, you may wobble reeling and fall. Plain and simple. The moderate breathing brings in more oxygen, which at that point clears out your organs, for example, the liver, which contains negative emotion, for example, grief, and outrage. The breathing and the poses, are individually done, which clears the stomach of gases, and stimulates blood flow. The inverted poses bring blood flow to your brain, which stimulates, and revitalizes your mind, your skin, your lungs, and assists in altering your temperament. The poses; open your middle and hips, which cause your heart to be open. When you change your physiology, from your fallback position, or shut, tight, and a seemingly monitored location, to an increasingly open area, your body begins to trick your mind. Gracious if I'm standing like this, I should not be depressed. If my chest is up, and my arms are out, possibly I'm upbeat, at any rate not pitiful. In the present moment, if you genuinely remain there, during the yoga pose, you realize that there is nothing from your life, which is happening right at this point. You are perfectly fine. If you snap your fingers; that snap is how quick, a present moment, zooms by. There is nothing worrisome, or that needs your immediate attention, no distracting voices, in your mind, that let you know are useless. It's merely you being mindful and doing a moderate, centered, yoga pose. Another element in a modified yoga class that helps give relief for depression is meditation. In pretty much all of the yoga classes, I put in meditation. Meditation, if practiced, enables clients to remain in the present moment, and furthermore allows them to detect, that they are adored, thought about, and there is a sheltered spot within. There is a wide range of sorts of meditation, including color meditation, question and answer meditation, open-eyed meditation, and so forth. At first, yoga takes a lot of centers and discipline. Modified yoga is a discipline, yet it's easier than a regular strenuous mat class. You practice the poses and the breathing, and your practice was NOT beating yourself up, and allowing yourself to acknowledge, that you are not perfect. When you create in yoga, your confidence additionally creates. Sometimes not far off, you realize, it was quite recently, that you couldn't do, a portion of the strength and conditioning, poses of yoga, and now you can. Earlier, you might not have had much karma, with balance, and now, you remain on one foot for 1 minute or more. The essential thing about a modified yoga class, since it's not as difficult as power yoga, is that everyone or nearly everyone can do some modified yoga. I have changed the mat and adjusted chair. You experience acceptance and not rejection, which makes you feel better about yourself. Self-acceptance is an essential element of clearing depression and anxiety. Self-acceptance enables you to recognize that you are not perfect, and hence, you don't need to DO everything perfect. You don't need to claim responsibility for others happiness, or their choices, that lead them to the unsatisfied spot, of their lives. Along these lines, if right now, you are struggling, with depression, anxiety, and suicidal considerations, get help. Some counseling can genuinely help and go to a restorative or modified yoga class. Not a yoga class, where everybody is very competitive, or the teacher drives you, past your limit. You need to go to a level, that you feel acceptance, respect, and regard, and that you are encouraged, to do, just what you can do, and whatever ability, or flexibility you accompany, you are encouraged. That class will be a transformational class for you! If you give it a shot, a modified yoga class alongside, that positive yoga teacher, will almost certainly assist you, in clearing depression and anxiety.

How to Turn Yourself Into a Super Brain With Super Brain Yoga
Need to improve your intelligence or even transform your children into super-people and encouraged with scholarships after scholarships? Here's a simple solution to your supplication...
Super Brain Yoga is one of the best methods of improving brain control. It's so simple to do, and yet its snappy viability has been entirely astonishing. This simple strategy can be clarified as pursues: While standing, hold our right ear with our left hand, with thumb contacting front side and index finger contacting posterior of the ear. At that point place our right hand to our left side ear in a similar manner. With our hands situated accurately in that capacity, at that point we're prepared to do the exercise part where we will do crouching or regular sit-up exercise. When going down, we have to inhale profoundly with stomach/mid-region,

and while getting up, we have to exhale slowly. The procedure of inhalation/exhalation ought to be secured inside the season of going down and getting up.

Entirely are 2 forms of relaxing:

- Breathing in a while in a while, hunching down and exhaling as you stand.
- Exhaling while at the same time hunching down and breathing in as you stand.

There's a video you can watch to enable you to all the more likely understand this simple and yet fantastic framework.

In Yoga custom, when the body bends forward, we exhale (breath out), and when the body stretches out, we inhale (breathe in. In this way, when we squat holding our ears with opposite hands, (our body bends forward) we exhale, and after standing back up, our body stretches, and along these lines, we inhale. This exercise has been credited with logical approval for its valuable impact of achieving entire all-encompassing brain (left and right brain) synchronization. This inclusive development must be performed slowly. Additionally, ensure that the eyes stay straight during the procedure for most significant advantages. Inhalation and exhalation should be possible as indicated by one's solace level, without causing torment nor uneasiness. The fundamental concern is to complete the inhalation and exhalation appropriately, that is all there's to it. A check of 14 to 21 redundancies for each day is beyond what enough and improvement can be found in 3 to about a month effectively. Some important precautionary measures to be pursued are:

1. Try to wear free pieces of clothing and be dressed serenely while playing out the exercise.

2. Ladies are not advised to do the exercise during periods, as it is accepted that "tainted vitality" living on the lower body may go up. Pregnant ladies are encouraged to counsel their doctor before endeavoring to play out this exercise every day.

3. The best time to do this exercise is in the early morning or later at night.

4. The better impact will be gotten when this is done on a void stomach.

5. Ensure the exercise is performed slowly for better outcomes.

Trust me; such a simple exercise can not just upgrade your intelligence and make you rationally fit, yet besides help you drop some additional pounds and be physically fit as well, not to mention disposing of the probability of contracting age-related diseases, for example, Parkinson's, and so forth. That is more than slaughtering 2 winged animals with one stone, as it were.

Training the Brain Through Sleep and Yoga
You, similar to your brain, is loaded with potential. We ought not to belittle ourselves and our brain.
Indeed, we live in a no-nonsense society, everything is going so quick, and we are besieged by such a significant number of components around us. Our brains can store and access the extraordinary heaps of data. In this way, we will, in general stress more and appreciate less. More often than not, we are too worn out to even think about relaxing our mind and have a decent rest! Rest is critical to general health and prosperity. At the point when individuals get under 6 or 7 hours of rest every night, their hazard for creating maladies starts to increment. Rest diminishes stress. A decent night's rest makes you feel stimulated and alert the following day. All the more significantly rest supports our memory. Memory consolidation happens during rest. While your body might rest, your brain is occupied with preparing your day, making associations between occasions, factual information, emotions, and recollections. Your fantasies and profound rest are a significant time for your brain to gain experiences and connections. Getting higher quality rest will enable you to recall and process things better. Things being what they are, how would we accomplish a decent night rest? The accompanying can perform great rest:

1. Listening to unwinding music
2. Avoiding before-bed snacks

3. Getting to bed right on time as could be allowed
4. Taking a hot shower or shower

Stress adds to memory decay. Another stress-reducer which I as of late began rehearsing is Yoga. Yoga is an incredible stress reducer. A couple of stretches every day is sufficient to discharge your physical pressure and trigger endorphins to make you feel good. Proficient use of the body cues movement in the brain. Yoga styles use specific meditation techniques to calm the mind.

The body and brain are accomplices! Also, Yoga offers this mind-body association. As you coordinate your controlled breathing with the movements of your body, you retrain your mind to find that spot of quiet and harmony. It additionally elevates improved flow to the brain too. Let us not misjudge ourselves. We have a great ability to learn. In contrast to PCs, our brain will never say: "Hard drive full." A great rest and yoga routine will release your mind's potential!

Why Brain Training?

The brain needs care only like the body.

New logical research demonstrates that we can improve the health and capacity of our brains with the privilege of mental exercises. In an examination subsidized by the National Institute of Health, researchers found that memory, thinking, and preparing pace can be improved by brain training. Additionally, they discovered that intellectual enhancement endured for in any event five years!

CHAPTER FOUR

Keeping Your Brain Working

We can help out our brains than we understand. What's more, the vast majority of what we can do are things that will help our general health too. For our brains and the health of our bodies, it is essential to remain hydrated, detoxified, and oxygenated. We can do this by drinking a lot of water. Green tea and peppermint tea are additionally a superb way to keep hydrated. Also, smoothies made with new leafy foods keep our brains stimulated. Having counts calories that comprise of an adequate supply of fish oil will boost our brain power. The familiar aphorism about an apple daily fending off the specialist isn't only a legend. They genuinely do support our brains and health. Salmon contains omega3 and protein for our bodies and brains; avocados increment bloodstream; arranged vegetables, especially those that are brilliantly hued, and natural product. Blueberries specifically are exceptionally painful. Different sustenances incorporate entire grains, olive oil, and cocoa, which will be good news for chocolate darlings to know. Important additionally is to have a generous breakfast and to maintain a strategic distance from greasy and sugary sustenances. Honest answers for kicking off your brain are to keep a diary; to take a stab at the composing verse, regardless of whether you figure you can't; listen to music and get your body going. Take a stab at learning an unknown dialect or an instrument. I'm giving the piano another attempt since my couple of exercises when I was eight years of age. It's stunning what I have recollected. Different ideas that are good for your brain and general prosperity are to think decidedly. There are always two ways of taking a gander at something. Why pick the negative form? Grin and snicker regularly. It will change your point of view on life. Keep socially dynamic and included. Listen to the ideas of others. They will give your brain a boost. Also, have you attempted to utilize chopsticks? That is positively an encounter. Exercise your memory. Invest energy with children, maybe play Wii with them or some other PC game. Take children on trips, converse with them, and truly listen to their perspectives on what they see and think. Children can carry on brilliant discussions, and you may find that it's a different way of taking a gander at life. They absolutely will make you think quicker. Play trivia recreations and if you don't progress admirably, make it a point to recall trivia facts. Keeping your brain dynamic can incorporate pastimes. What are yours? Are you perusing, weaving, photography, water hues, yoga, or reflection? Physical exercise is right for your brain, your body, and your general health. Don't stop excessively near your goal with the goal that you have a further separation from walking. Take the stairs rather than the lift, do yard work, walk the pooch, swim, move, and play golf. Most things you accomplish for your brain will likewise support your body and increment your general feeling of prosperity. With that, life turns out to be progressively pleasant. Sylvia Behnish has distributed 'Rollercoaster Ride With Brain Injury (For Loved Ones)', a genuine book specifying the troublesome year following a brain injury; 'His Sins', a three-generation family saga about how the activities of one individual can influence who and what is to come, and 'Life's Challenges, A Short Story Collection'.

Tips to Control Your Brain
You can expand the capacity of your brain to hold and imitate information. You can likewise guarantee that your memory stays active till cutting edge age.
Hippocampus is that part of the brain that screens all form of reviewing including the long haul ones. Wellbeing researchers at Virginia University in America concentrating this central zone of the human brain have thought of a startling revelation that we once in a while start measures to deal with our brain. In straightforward words, we underestimate this vital organ of our body - the brain. As a part of their inquiries about, the specialists have discovered that memory can blur, and furthermore this fatal disorder can strike an individual when she/he is in the mid-twenties. This issue is named as 'blurring memory.' It has additionally been seen that an individual can assimilate any information, help the pace of dissects and settling issues or riddles - activities the brain is included with - before achieving the age of

30. The, for the most part, goes down after the 27 years old. Don't be harried! It doesn't happen all the time with all type of people. In any case, it happens with people who infrequently use their capacity to adjust their brains.

The best part of these tips is that they can be polished at home or even in your office; they are very prudent too.

Consequently, scientists have concocted the accompanying tips to make your brain ever youthful...

THE STRATEGY

The mantra is to keep up an evergreen brain in a solid body. Resolve pressure, and go for unwinding.

PLAY MIND GAMES

The more you keep your brain active by playing different types of fixation, including games, the more productive will your brain remain. Get taken on club activities where you will be required to make such games with the individuals.

Your memory is industriously burdened to stay alert. All the while, your brain is restored, and your memory is tried while you are engaged. Stress-busting psychological distractions are chess, memory testing card games, just as some computer games. You can play solo or in gathering.

Train yourself to recollect numbers orchestrated in different ways or names of people or even the vehicle numbers as they cruise by. Mental prompts are a must. You can advance your strategies.

REMAIN PHYSICALLY FIT

An active body can be conceivable just when you have the right diet with adequate calories. Physical and mental exercises enhance this wholesome diet. You can decide on yoga or other active forms of freehand or practice center connected calendars. Yoga offers adaptability to the appendages while the reflection part of it builds focus. The consolidated impact is that the brain is siphoned with oxygenated blood. The recreation center exercises set your adrenalin streaming too. All forms of activities that get your blood streaming are perfect for your brain as well. Cycling, swimming, and running can be great ways of keeping your body, psyche, and brain active and kicking. NOTE: The ideal way to go about everything is to look for the guidance of your doctor. This is significant as our bodies need time to conform to the new timetables of exercises. Try not to go for a feverish or overactive exercise routine if you have had a somewhat laid-back program generally. Else, the sudden move in the day by day schedule can be unsafe.

Wholesome diet

What we eat has a particular state on what we do with our brains. This is fundamental because relying upon our diet, our hearts work. Thus, pick green and new food things. Guarantee that your body gets all forms of supplements from the dishes that you devour. There must be an adequate measure of Omega-3 unsaturated fats. Always vote in favor of a diet that is wealthy in cancer prevention agent: incorporate pecans, carrots, and almonds.

These solutions mean saying a definite "NO!" to quick and lousy nourishment. Also, avoid food that contains additives.

Top 10 Way to Train Your Brain For Peak Performance
Numerous individuals have issues with recalling things such forgot where you put your keys? Can't recollect phone numbers? Or on the other hand, forgot where you left your car. So you're not the only one truly on this issue, but instead, there are great ways that you can use to improve your memory. Here are 10 ways, which you can pursue to keep your memory fit as a fiddle, and furthermore techniques that can assist you with improving your memory's condition and performance.

1. Eat your brain food

What we eat each day affects the performance and long-haul condition of our memory. Reviews in recent decades have appeared certain foods can contribute to the better functioning of the neural circuits of the brain that control memory. Fish and foods that contain a lot of omega oils support the brain, and this can help improve your memory. Include a lot of leafy foods in your eating routine and stay away from foods that are high in sugar.

2. Physical exercise

Physical exercise increases the progression of oxygen and nutrients in the blood. The advantages of exercise affect emphatically many body frameworks, and particularly our memory and other cognitive capabilities. It is sufficient to exercise for 20 minutes every day in straightforward types of use such as strolling, cycling, swimming, and dancing.

3. Make A Showing

Play connects with the prefrontal cortex, in charge of your most abnormal amount cognitive functions - including self-learning, memory, mental symbolism, and incentive and reward processing. Activities like extension, chess, sudoku, pretending recreations and challenging crossword confuse all give thorough neural exercises.

4. Reflect

Reflection is an excellent way to focus your mind and stir your brain toward the beginning of the day. Make an opportunity to sit and intervene for 15 minutes each morning, focusing on just your breath and heartbeat. Your intercession session will leave you feeling calm and ready to start creating your day. Intervene again before bed to let your mind normally filter through the leftovers of the day and set yourself up for a restful rest.

5. Music

Music is an excellent exercise for the mind. Tuning in to the right sort of music will enable your brain to process information better and become progressively receptive to that information. Tuning in to classical music composed by Mozart or Beethoven is exceedingly recommended.

6. Get a lot of rest.

A few scientists accept that the poor rest examples and lack of sleep experienced by many exhausted grown-ups - contribute to absentmindedness and memory misfortune. Go for in any event at least 7 hours of rest each night to keep your brain functioning getting it done.

7. Learn constantly

Search for topics that interest you and genuinely engage with adapting new information and advancements about them. Consider something that you've always needed to figure out how to do and afterward begin. Perusing, following lectures, programs, information on TV and the Internet, are sources of continuous education for your brain with beneficial outcomes to your memory.

8. Reduce Stress
When you're Stress or restless, you can't concentrate or process information. Figure out how to calm yourself with breathing exercises. Yoga offers a great way to loosen up. Remind yourself of what's significant and exceptional in your life. Release its rest.

9. Take a vitamin
Vitamin and nutrients invigorate the functioning of the brain and are beneficial in memory maintenance. Specific vitamins assume an essential job in brain wellbeing and memory, including B-vitamins, choline, vitamin E, vitamin C, Omega-3 Fatty Acids, and other cancer prevention agent nutrients.

10. Fragrance based treatment
Studies show fragrance-based treatment can be utilized for both the body and the mind, facilitating physical and enthusiastic ailments and improve the state of mind, memory, and concentration. One herb that mainly helps the brain is rosemary.

Meditation Can Improve Your Brain Function
If you've effectively taken a stab at yoga, at that point, you may likewise have dunked your toe into the universe of meditation. It's incredible stuff and not only for individuals who develop pot and eat only crude natural products. It's something that I attempt to do ordinarily as it's something that keeps me grounded and quiet. It likewise assists with my instinct and inward certainty. As of late, someone in the scholarly world - specifically the University of Wisconsin - saw that meditation isn't only some 'novel' practice. However, it has incredible potential. A relevant report presumed that meditation could decrease pressure, help with

insusceptibility, and even assistance your brain to work better. Who might have imagined that just by contemplating for a couple of minutes consistently, you'd probably advantage from such a significant number of outcomes?

The most effective method to do it. It's not hard to do, and if you need to attempt it for yourself, at that point, you should sit serenely. Next, close your eyes and concentrate on your breathing. Feel the air as it leaves behind your noses and into your lungs. Do it again and focus on the goal that you can do it slower and more profound. Whatever musings you get, at that point see them yet given them a chance to pass. Maintain your attention on your breathing. At the point when your mind meanders, bring it back and refocus on your breath. When you've done this for 10 to 15 minutes - at that point you've effectively meditated. Discover different projects for assortment. There is a lot of data online about how to meditate. For instance, there are sites, writes, and even podcasts that give direction on alternative ways to meditate. A portion of the styles will take you on an inward pictured journey that will leave you feeling revived and restored. Have a go at making a gander at the podcasts for iPhone for this sort of substance. Allows return to that research for a minute, as there's something else in there that is intriguing. The University of Wisconsin attempted one of the outcomes from this research, was that meditation is as useful for your brain as your body. The researchers up there concentrated some accomplished meditators and found that they had more generation of gamma brain waves. These waves have a relationship with more transparent and increasingly centered reasoning. These gamma waves weren't merely in real life during the time the meditation was assuming taking the position - they were there nonstop. They additionally found that there was not the typical age-related diminishing in the zone of the brain that is utilized for consideration and tactile observation. This is all uplifting news for us all. It implies that we can keep dynamic rationally and physically for more, and this can go towards delaying our wellbeing into our later years. Goodness and one more thing that you should know as well. Only 40 minutes of meditation can complete much more for you rationally with regards to being alert than a 40-minute catnap can. Having a snooze can make you feel lethargic for as long as an hour a while later. However, you won't have to endure that if you supplant the ZZZs with some meditation. So with the majority of that proof, it would seem that meditation is, at last, being perceived for its forces. It will ensure you against the adverse outcomes of being pushed and tense, and it will bolster

How to Switch Off and Relax When Your Brain Is Busy
What would you be able to do if your brain won't switch off, or is excessively loaded with stuff for you to relax?
It isn't always awful to have lots of stuff circumventing your head. Once in a while, you need to invoke new thoughts or solutions to issues. However, when your brain winds up insane with musings that you can't switch off, what do you do?

- It's hard to relax after work.
- It's hard to ponder anything.
- You can't concentrate.
- You feel like you need to shout or run away.

What's more, it can cause tension in your body just as headaches. What you truly need to do is locate the off switch, which is way actually quite tricky.

Some straightforward solutions to relax and switch your brain off are:

- Medication
- an absorb the shower
- be whimsical and run around accomplishing something idiotic for some time
- yoga or judo
- a treatment, for example, rub
- Another diversion where you are compelled to concentrate on something explicitly, such as adopting new move ventures for example

Be that as it may, imagine a scenario where these exercises neglect to enable you to relax.

Now and then people will go after a beverage, have another cigarette, over enjoy chocolate, or any number of not precisely accommodating propensities. I don't think this is hugely a solution. I would suggest some vitality work. For me, I call it Reiki, yet any mending from a recommended expert or companion will do it. (I trust it's everything similar stuff from the same spot.)

You may ask why this is superior to anything the various proposals I made. Well, I have been utilizing Reiki since 1997, and I have found that it has an unusual way of finding the off switch for your brain. I know - I didn't think there was one either.

Here are two stories that delineate my point.

One night I was lying in bed, yet I wasn't attempting to sleep. I was frantically trying to recollect the thing that I neglected to record that was hugely significant for me to do the following day. I rationally experienced my daily agenda, yet I can't floating off and beginning to nod off. At that point, I understood that my accomplice's hand was laying all around delicately on the highest point of my head. I went to him and stated, 'For what reason is your hand on my head?' Consequently, he stated, 'I thought you were experiencing difficulty getting the chance to sleep, so I thought I'd give you some Reiki.' That is the reason I couldn't think! My brain was switching off! Flook? You may think so however things like that have happened way too often. Here's another story. I was taking an interest in an open day for a yoga focus where I was allowing people 10-minute sessions of Reiki to experience it. It wasn't perfect, there wasn't room for a mentor, so I had a chair at the edge of the room, and a lot a more significant number of people turned up than foreseen. So when somebody was sat in the chair having Reiki people were strolling past them, directly alongside them. I continued reasoning this couldn't in any way, shape, or form be relaxing, and I was somewhat stressed over it that they wouldn't get the best experience. Nobody said anything to me regarding this until a man came up to talk. He wasn't generally in to 'so much stuff' as he put it, he had quite recently flown in with his better half. Be that as it may, he suspected he'd have a take a quick trip and see what this 'Reiki' thing was about while he was hanging tight for her. There he sat for ten minutes having some Reiki with me stressing that it wouldn't be relaxing, and he unmistakably didn't get it anyway so most likely wouldn't have an incredible experience. At the point when the ten minutes was up, I set my hand on his shoulder and delicately instructed him to take his mindfulness back to the room. He opened his eyes and looked very doubtful. I inquired as to whether he was okay and would be like a glass of water. He said he was okay he just pondered when everybody had returned as he hadn't heard them. 'What do you mean?' I answered. What's more, he stated, 'Soon after you began everybody left, where did they go? I expected there was a showing in another room or something. However, I didn't hear them return, and when I opened my eyes, they were all back'. No, I clarified, nobody had gone anyplace, in certainty more people had arrived and kept on strolling past him, pretty intently, for the entire ten minutes. He looked like he genuinely didn't trust me yet said that he did for sure feel extremely relaxed. These are just two out of numerous models regarding why I think Reiki, or comparable, will genuinely assist you with switching off and appropriately relax when your brain is humming, you are on edge, or have lots at the forefront of your thoughts. Furthermore, in the event that you genuinely need to take advantage of it, and of life, yourself and the universe, I would exceedingly propose that you learn Reiki for yourself, it's not tied in with offering medications to other people, it's in a general sense a self-improvement instrument and will totally change your reality if you let it.

CHAPTER FIVE

Tips To Increase Your Brain Powers

The brain is a little yet most powerful organ of the body that controls all our thinking, sentiments, activities, feelings, and considerably more. This small organ is comprised of billions of neurons that develop with proper diet and exercise. Your prosperity mainly relies upon the sharpness of your mind, improved memory, and thinking abilities. Deal with your brain and appreciate a fruitful life.

I am giving underneath specific tips that will push you to build your brain powers generously:

1. Eat Brain Healthy Foods

A few foods are especially useful for the brain which you should incorporate into your diet, for example, fish, eggs, green vegetables, tomatoes, broccoli, blueberries, entire grains, almonds, pecans, peanuts and pumpkin seeds. Stay away from alcoholic and carbonated beverages instead drink plain water and green tea.

2. Deal with Your Overall Fitness

The health of our brain is uniquely identified with our general wellness. The brain stays healthy in a healthy body. Physical exercise isn't suitable for your body yet besides your brain. Do whatever exercise you like, for example, walking, running, swimming, heart stimulating exercise, yoga and so forth., yet do it regularly.

3. Meditation and Deep Breathing

Meditation is an excellent method for loosening up your body and mind in this manner, expanding your brain powers. A few people do meditation for looking for profound edification while others accomplish for internal harmony and tranquility. Continuously do meditation in a quiet and calm spot. Be that as it may, you can do deep breathing whenever and at wherever. Aside from the various health advantages of a deep breath, it is likewise useful for the development of brain cells.

4. Get Enough Sleep

The vast majority overlook the significance of a pleasant evening's sleep. The absence of sleep can seriously hurt the working of the brain. If you feel that your mind is clear or sleepy, then it implies that you needest. Head to sleep and sleep. Take enough sleep day by day and see your brain working much better because sleep enables your brain to merge and sort out data. Additionally, taking a 15-20 minutes nap during the day can hone your mind and improve your essential leadership powers.

5. Peruse and Write

Perusing and composing are good propensities and very accommodating in expanding the brain powers. Keep some good books in your bedroom and read a couple of pages before resting. Likewise work on composing, in any event, a couple of sentences, on another theme each day.

6. Think Positively

Stress, uneasiness, depression, and negative thinking are the principle guilty parties of devastating the brain nerve cells. Dispose of all sort of pessimism from your mind, beyond what many would consider possible. Build up the propensity for seeing the bright side of things. Positive thinking is a method for carrying on with a happy life.

7. Give Task To Your Brain

Give your brain the undertaking of tackling fundamental issues, puzzles and crosswords, and so forth. The more you use your brain, the more the brain cells will develop. In any case, keep away from over thinking and performing various tasks. Complete one thing at a time and don't overweight your mind with different errands.

8. Love Nature

It is always useful to invest some energy in a typical habitat. Go to the mountains, walk in the wilderness, do drifting in the streams, sit by the side of the lake, and value the encompassing normal magnificence. Nature revives your mind and heart. Sitting in a characteristic encompassing and breathing deeply removes all your depression and fortifies your brain muscles.

Other TIPS

An ongoing issue of a magazine incorporates a rundown of 10 activities to help your brain health. The review includes numerous activities I would call crucial for general wellbeing. In this aggressive condition, there is a propensity to overlook health and spotlight seriously on a pursuit of employment or occupation. It is essential to make a stride back and ensure that we are dealing with ourselves, as well. You might need to attempt a couple of these 10 activities: .

Add assortment to your life. Try not to pursue a set schedule without fail. Wake up your brain with something new. Attempt another course to the workplace. Go to another systems administration gathering. Retain another poem.

Be a Life Long Learner. Study something inside and out. This is good for your brain and your career. Get familiar with another dialect and start to talk and compose it. (I just began an impromptu creation class which is good for my brain and fun!)

Tackle Puzzles/Play games - Try crossword puzzles, Sudoku, connect as well as chess. They recommend attempting to finish before time runs out because that rouses snappier thinking. In my comedy class games, we need to think about a word on the beat of a musicality begun by the educator. It is difficult. However, you improve at it with training. Reminds me of a Miss Mary Mac, a game I played as a kid.

Clear the mind - Use meditation, yoga, or a walk in the forested areas to help clear your mind. The more significant part of us has active thoughts today. A portion of the prattle is loud and harmful. It is essential to set aside an effort to clear your mind regularly. While you are busy, take some deep breaths to scrub your mind and body. Get 8 hours sleep a night - Your brain needs a rest as well. This is the time for it to unite the day's recollections. Give your brain time to do this by getting an entire eight hours of sleep. Bunches of research shows people in the US don't get enough sleep!

Be creative - Use your creative mind each day. Set aside the effort to paint, add to your diary, make another site, compose a poem, or do whatever uses the right (creative) side of your brain.

Invest energy with friends - Staying without anyone else's input all the time can put your brain into log jam mode. (Performances know.) Friends, family, and partners help keep you occupied with life, and that keeps your brain dynamic and working. Being agreeable is right for your brain and your soul. People with a robust network of friends and colleagues live more and more joyful lives all in all. (Systems administration is right for your brain!)

Eat a proper diet - Include foods grown from the ground in your diet alongside entire grains and fish. My folks used to disclose to me fish was brain food. I surmise they were correct!!

Have regular check-ups with the specialist - Blood weight, glucose, weight, cholesterol all are important to proper brain work. Ensure yours are in the typical range and if not work with your specialist to get them under tight restraints.

Keep Your Brain Healthy

Much the same as it is vital for us to deal with our bodies, it is essential to deal with our brains also. You fuel your body with healthy foods and exercise. You can form and characterize your muscles, and free or put on weight to change your appearance. So what would you be able to do to deal with your brain? Here are ten things to do to kick you off. Pursue these ten stages to deal with your brain, and you may find that you are a superior understudy, you may even learn something!

1. Work it out

Your brain needs exercise the same amount of as your body does. It is workable for your brain to decay only like your muscles. You can exercise your brain by making it think. Make your brain feel by completing a crossword puzzle or play a word game with a friend. Peruse a fascinating book, (perusing is a major one), watch a however inciting motion picture and get inventive with a pastime. These things can stimulate and work your brain, making it capacity better. If you are experiencing considerable difficulties with homework or a task, have a go at taking a break and completing one of these things.

2. Get Going!

Our bodies flourish with physical exercise, even our brains. When you exercise, your heart works more diligently to siphon the blood through your body, expanding oxygenation in your brain, which is, as it were, practicing your brain. It is an excellent plan to go on a walk in the middle of classes or enjoy a reprieve from homework to exercise to get your mind working.

3. Challenge Yourself!

Learning new things makes new roads in your brain and challenges it. When you learn new data, your brain ends up healthier. Take a stab at learning something new, go to a cooking class, or learn yoga. Play chess with a friend or travel; after all, "travel expands the mind." It is essential to learn new things always for the health of our brains.

4. Eat Brain Foods

Truly, they exist. Brain foods will be foods that give essential nutrients to your brain. Most importantly, always begin your day off with a good breakfast. Eating breakfast awakens you and gives you the nutrients you have to begin thinking and working. Studies demonstrate that people that have breakfast devour fewer calories for the day and have higher working digestion also. Foods brimming with cell reinforcements like blueberries, and pomegranate are suitable for your brain alongside fish, avocado, fruits and vegetables, and entire grains.

5. Vitamins

Your mother always instructed you to take your vitamins, and she was correct. Your brain blossoms with the nutrients in vitamins and enhancements so make beyond any doubt that you are placing them into your body. Omega-3, vitamin B, E and C, grape seed concentrate and a lot of water are just a couple of the things that you ought to be mindfully adding to your eating routine to keep a healthy brain.

6. Avoid, Avoid, Avoid

There is a restriction on all things. Much the same as there are good things for your brain, there are likewise terrible things for your brain. For example, medications and liquor can murder brain cells. You ought to likewise avoid or use with some restraint substances like caffeine, hydrogenated vegetable oils, intensely handled foods, and fast foods. What's more, last yet surely not least, don't smoke. Cigarette smoking burglarizes your brain of oxygen and can cause numerous issues. Indeed, there are concentrates out there that connection some Alzheimer's patients to tobacco.

7. Ensure your Noggin

Shielding your brain from damage is unquestionably one way to keep it healthy and keen. Mishaps, including your brain can be wrecking to the idea that your brain capacities. Always wear a protective cap and wear a safety belt. Be careful when playing physical games like football and rugby. Redundant wounds to the brain can cause substantial harm that can't be fixed.

8. Relax

Stress can be tough on your brain. It is to your most significant advantage to diminish importance however much as could be expected for your mind and your body. Decreasing stress can likewise improve your mental health and condition of prosperity. In case you have a feeling that you're near the edge, attempt to cut the stress levels down a score. Watch an amusing motion picture, take a walk or scrub down. Be sure and have a fabulous time do whatever it takes not to give stress a chance to cut you down and your brain will be significantly happier.

9. Stimulate your Senses

Fragrant healing, knead, working in a greenhouse, and preparing are everything that can stimulate your senses and influence your brain. At the point when your brain is exposed to multi-sensory activities stimulates your brain and helps keep your mind sharp. For example, when you prepare treats, you consolidate the fixings, manipulate the mixture, and smell the treats.

10. Be a Social Butterfly

Your brain is stimulated when you converse with friends and family. When you share experiences and feelings, your brain gets stimulants that it needs. Having and making friends is additionally useful for your mental health. Sentiments of confinement and forlornness vanish when you encircle yourself with friends and family.

7 Tips How to Perk Up Your Brain
For certain people, awakening and leaving their comfortable beds is a great gallant deed. Be that as it may, when you complete one act, it is simpler to do the following. How would you make your brain wake up with you? Here are 7 working ways to perk up your brain.

1. Physical exercises.
Physical exercises keep your body fit as a fiddle as well as keep your brain working, as because of the escalated developments, the blood flows better in your body just as in your brain. The best exercises for awakening your brain are ones when your head is arranged lower your heart (there are numerous positions like this in yoga).

2. Drink water, not coffee.
Many looks into demonstrate that coffee doesn't influence our productivity as extraordinary as everybody might suspect. A glass of water can complete a greatly improved activity that will last more. Water on an empty stomach initiates the work of gastrointestinal tract, yet doesn't disturb mucous film as coffee does.

3. Various flavors can make you concentrate better.
Principle speaking, people don't recognize great. Although scents can enable you to concentrate and brighten you up. The experts recommend utilizing scents of basil, rosemary, Melissa, rose, and lavender.

4. Optimism in everything.
It's anything but a mystery that each work, particularly savvy one, goes better in quiet air. It isn't always conceivable to make such an air, however. Be that as it may, if you learn how to concentrate your consideration on the splendid sides, your productivity will increment.

5. Puzzles.
A good exercise for your brain will unravel different crossword puzzles, problems, riddles, and so forth.

6. Healthy eating.
The ideal way to clear mind and a good memory is healthy eating that comprises of fruits and vegetables. You can eat some chocolate once in a while. It is likewise perfect for your brain.

7. Never quit learning something.
Regardless of whether the most brilliant mind quits being dynamic, it will become dull soon. That is the reason you have to prepare it always. Learn unknown dialect, learn how to draw, cook, and so on 15-minute brain exercises, every day can anticipate any corruption.

How to Perk Up Your Brain

Top 3 Tips to Care For Your Lungs, Heart and Brain
Much the same as it is significant for us to deal with our bodies, it is essential to deal with our brains also. You fuel your body with healthy foods and exercise. You can form and characterize your muscles, and free or put on weight to change your appearance. So what would you be able to do to deal with your brain? Here are ten things to do to kick you off. Pursue these ten stages to deal with your brain, and you may find that you are a superior understudy, you may even learn something!

1. Work it out
Your brain needs exercise the same amount of as your body does. It is feasible for your brain to decay only like your muscles. You can exercise your brain by making it think. Make your brain feel by completing a crossword perplex or play a word game with a friend. Peruse a fascinating book, (perusing is a major one), watch a however inciting film and get innovative with a side interest. These things can invigorate and work your brain, making it capacity better. If you are experiencing considerable difficulties with

homework or a task, have a go at taking a break and completing one of these things.

2. Get Going!

Our bodies blossom with physical exercise, even our brains. When you exercise, your heart works more earnestly to siphon the blood through your body, expanding oxygenation in your brain, which is, as it were, practicing your brain. It is an excellent plan to go on a walk in the middle of classes or enjoy a reprieve from homework to exercise to get your mind working.

3. Challenge Yourself!

Learning new things makes new roads in your brain and difficulties it. When you learn new data, your brain winds up healthier. Take a stab at learning something new, go to a cooking class, or learn yoga. Play chess with a friend or travel, after all, "travel widens the mind." It is imperative to learn new things always for the health of our brains.

4. Eat Brain Foods

Indeed, they exist. Brain foods will be foods that give vital nutrients to your brain. As a matter of first importance always begin your vacation day with a good breakfast. Having breakfast awakens you and gives you the nutrients you have to start thinking and working. Studies demonstrate that individuals that have breakfast expend fewer calories for the day and have higher working digestion also. Foods loaded with cell reinforcements like blueberries, and pomegranate is right for your brain alongside fish, avocado, leafy foods, and entire grains.

5. Vitamins

Your mother always instructed you to take your vitamins, and she was correct. Your brain flourishes with the nutrients in vitamins and enhancements so make beyond any doubt that you are placing them into your body. Omega-3, vitamin B, E and C, grape seed concentrate and a lot of water are just a couple of the things that you ought to be mindfully adding to your eating regimen to keep a healthy brain.

6. Dodge, Avoid, Avoid

There is a restriction on all things. Much the same as there are good things for your brain, there are additionally awful things for your brain. For example, medications and liquor can slaughter brain cells. You ought to likewise dodge or use with some restraint substances like caffeine, hydrogenated vegetable oils, vigorously handled foods and fast foods. Furthermore, last yet unquestionably not least, don't smoke. Cigarette smoking loots your brain of oxygen and can cause numerous issues. Indeed, there are concentrates out there that connection some Alzheimer's patients to tobacco.

7. Ensure your Noggin

Shielding your brain from damage is unquestionably one way to keep it healthy and brilliant. Mishaps, including your brain, can be decimating to the idea that your brain capacities. Always wear a protective cap and wear a safety belt. Be careful when playing physical games like football and rugby. Redundant wounds to the brain can cause substantial harm that can't be fixed.

8. Relax

Stress can be tough on your brain. It is to your most significant advantage to lessen stress however much as could reasonably be expected for your mind and your body. Reducing stress can likewise improve your mental health and condition of prosperity. In case you incline that you're near the edge, attempt to cut the stress levels down a score. Watch an entertaining film, take a walk or wash up. Be sure and have a fabulous time do whatever it takes not to give stress a chance to cut you down and your brain will be significantly happier.

9. Invigorate your Senses

Fragrance based treatment, rub, working in a nursery, and heating is everything that can animate your faculties and impact your brain. At the point when your brain is exposed to multi-tactile exercises energizes your brain and helps keep your mind sharp. For example, when you prepare treats, you consolidate the fixings, massage the batter, and smell the treats.

10. Be a Social Butterfly

Your brain is animated when you converse with friends and family. When you offer encounters and feelings, your brain gets stimulants that it needs. Having and making friends is additionally useful for your mental health. Sentiments of separation and depression vanish when you encircle yourself with friends and family.

Your Brain on Yoga: Proven Positive Impacts

At this point, it's turned out to be clear to most that practicing yoga goes a long way past having long, lean appendages and impeccable stance. It is winding up increasingly clear that yoga is extremely a way of life. Along these lines of life begins in the studio, yet has a fantastic way of penetrating all aspects of your reality by hacking into your brain and changing the way you manage different situations. In this manner, yoga moves toward becoming not what we do; however, how we do it. Yoga is the practice of syncing breath with development, resisting the urge to panic while doing a testing movement. This is the reason for the dramatic change that happens in our brains when we practice. While we practice, we re-align the way we experience emotions, for example, stress, depression, and tension, by taking advantage of the systems that make those emotions and changing the furrows in our brains. Regardless of what the situation might be, whether it's running from a tiger or taking a last, most crucial test, the sensory system has one reaction to stress. This includes muscle tenseness, shortness of breath, negative considerations, and the arrival of cortisol into the circulation system. When we stay formed and control our breath while putting our body into awkward positions, such as completing a headstand or winding into spun bound half-moon, the brain gets reinvented to react proactively and to stay loose in a stressful situation. This action truly hacks the brain by setting off specific emotions and after that revamping our common reactions. Taken far enough, this empowers us to take advantage of the most astounding potential working of our creatures to accomplish whatever objective we put forward.

When we figure out how to diminish self-judgment and dread through yoga, the conceivable outcomes of life open up and all

that we want and need winds up charged towards us. The practice of falling all over attempting to do flying pigeon or lifting your leg one inch higher in the third warrior tells your brain that your questions don't control you. By going towards vulnerability and uneasiness in our stances, we register that our apprehensions of what will happen to exist as impediments, and naturally have no power or legitimacy. By practicing yoga, we not just sculpt our bodies, we carve our psyches and saddle the extraordinary power we hold inside. Go forward in confidence towards your practice, and realize that each battle is in the most astounding enthusiasm of your body, psyche, and soul.
With Great Love and Unlimited Possibilities!!

Exercise May Be The Fountain Of Youth For Your Brain
Alright, I get it. Not very many of us genuinely need to bounce up and hit the treadmill or go to the gym. You did make that New Year's goals, isn't that right? You guaranteed yourself you would get fit as a fiddle and get healthier. Furthermore, what will that exercise accomplish for you? It may not be a genuine wellspring of youth. You want all of a sudden level your mid-region and consume 15 pounds, yet a regular exercise routine during the time will be a standout amongst the best things you accomplish for yourself. What's more, it will improve your body, yet additionally your brain.

Memory
Keep in mind how you overlook everything? No? Well, one problem might be that you don't get enough exercise for the day. The hippocampus, the piece of the brain in charge of learning and memory functions, reacts well to cardiovascular and high-impact aerobics. In studies of the two kids and grown-ups, specialists found that the hippocampus developed as the members turned out to be progressively fit. In different studies, more seasoned adults demonstrated a similar connection between movement and brain structure changes. Momentary studies have additionally shown that increased physical movement can lead to better learning and memory functions. One German study took a gander at how members took in a language. After consistently strolling or cycling during unknown dialect learning, test subjects were better

ready to review vocabulary words.

Creativity

Everyone has innovative droops. Scholars, choreographers, even mathematicians frequently search for imaginative answers for dynamic problems. While inertia can lead to one robust finished method for moving toward challenges, exercise has been shown to support creativity with regards to tending to specific issues. Understudies at Stanford University intended to test this theory and walked around the school grounds. They encountered an increase in the quantity of free-wandering thought they had. They were better ready to deal with related academic problems. Unfaltering strolling helps quiet the nerves, and it advances creativity.

Degenerative Conditions

We don't more often than not consider Parkinson's sickness. We are beginning to ponder Alzheimer's. Both are certain degenerative neurological conditions that many are probably going to create before the finish of their lives. The science is still somewhat insecure on the issue on the precise causes. In any case, there is some examination that focuses on eating less and exercise commitments. Studies have shown that exercise will delay, if not avoid, the beginning of dementia. Also, you don't need to kill yourself in the gym, 30 to 40 minutes of strolling three to five times each week can altogether decrease your risk. What's more, it's not just the vigorous exercises that help. Equalization, opposition or weight training exercise, and yoga additionally help. One study watching German seniors who rehearsed yoga lifted weights in static positions and went out even two times per week saw increased brain cell connections. This was astonishment as it was recently felt that individuals of this age could never again fabricate more up to date and more grounded brain structures. Exercise lessens insulin obstruction and aggravation, the main drivers of numerous health problems. One of the exercises' extraordinary blessings is the incitement of growth factors that advance brain cell health. Regular practice develops recruits vessel growth and supports the growth and survival of new brain cells. Last, exercise encourages increase oxygen levels to the brain. This improves mental execution. It likewise moderates the rate of weakness, recovers generally speaking brain function, upgrades motor skills, and invigorates better bloodstream all through the body. By implication, exercise manages problems that add to intellectual hindrance, by boosting disposition, advancing better rest, diminishing pressure and bringing down uneasiness. It's honestly not about what you do as much as it is that you accomplish something. Everything necessary is a thirty minutes stroll through a recreation center. Not exclusively will you feel altogether better; however, you will modify your brain structure and function. That will enable you to recollect data for a test, your activity, whatever, and you'll lessen your risk of creating certain degenerative brain infections.

CHAPTER SIX

Brain Fitness Games

You're grinding away, acquainting another representative with an associate, and you immediately overlook their name. Or on the other hand, you go to the supermarket to get something "critical," and you erratically meander the aisles attempting to recall for what reason you're there. Sound well-known? As we age, we, for the most part, find our brains feeling less and less dependable in our daily lives, and sooner or later, maybe we cross a limit and immediately stress this may be a pattern. Be that as it may, the official inquiry is: What would we be able to do to keep our brains sharp? There are numerous things we can do to challenge our brains. We could select ourselves in a propelled math course, or read the Webster's Unabridged Dictionary from front to back; however, neither of those decisions is by all accounts uniquely engaging. Another choice is to play any of the developing numbers of brain fitness games that are springing up in a variety of areas, including on the web, CDs and DVDs, and even game consoles. In case you accomplish something healthy, you should have a good time simultaneously. Brain fitness games have a strong establishment in science and offer a changed and complex exercise over numerous areas of the brain. Although these games depend on science to be powerful, for them to pick up mainstream acknowledgment, they should likewise be conveyed in an engaging and drawing in way. Casual gaming standards are an ideal fit, as they are designed to be fun and open to differing audiences, including those that are new to gaming. The commitment and clean of a well-designed brain game not just can intrigue an enormous statistic; however, can likewise enable players to find the motivation to exercise their brains regularly.

Brain Fitness and Casual Gaming
The unstable development of gaming keeps on bringing a lot of decent variety into the industry, including new sorts, dissemination models, platforms, and info gadgets. Subsequently,

the statistic keeps on extending, making more open doors in areas that were recently viewed as excessively little or specialty to achieve the mainstream. With classification making titles like The Brain Age, Wii Fit and Guitar Hero appreciating blockbuster deals, an ever increasing number of people that haven't generally believed themselves to be "gamers" are getting actively engaged with games on a regular basis, which isn't only extraordinary for the current industry, yet in addition for new organizations and plans of action that push the limits of what we at present allude to as "games". There is a large section of the casual audience, for the most part in the child of post-war America statistic, who appreciate occasional game substance yet didn't grow up with games, and subsequently, don't feel that games offer enough an incentive to be a regular piece of their daily lives. Nonetheless, the ongoing flood of wellbeing-focused games has created new enthusiasm, bringing more people into games and moving the observation that games offer just entertainment. Brain fitness games specifically are an incredible fit for these casual audiences, as the 30+ group that makes up the center occasional statistic, is additionally bound to think about the significance of keeping the mind sharp, for their regular day to day existences, just as their future. The online space, without hardly lifting a finger of access to such a large number of people, is the ideal spot for people to play fun, tough games that animate the brain, and even feel that it's an essential utilization of their time.

Reinforcing the Mind by Increasing "Brain Reserve"
One of the fundamental ideas at the center of brain fitness is the idea of "brain reserve", additionally identified with the concept of brain versatility, which can be reinforced at about any point of individual's life by doing errands that are novel and complex, and invigorate a fair variety of areas inside the brain. Brain reserve identifies with the brain's ability to physically redesign itself in light of the requests set upon it. A brain with a healthy reserve is one that has shaped numerous cellular connections and is wealthy in brain cell thickness. A healthy reserve is by and abundant accepted to be able to defer the beginning of mental disintegration, for example, Alzheimer's Disease (AD). Mental illnesses must work longer and harder to show in a brain that has developed an active

reserve. A healthy brain should resemble a lavish and lively wilderness, as opposed to an island with a single palm tree. A desert like a brain is illustrative of a healthy brain, since it is loaded with cellular connections that are incredibly thick, and along these lines show a solid brain reserve. If you consider mental sickness like AD as a weed-whacker, it attacks the brain and starts to do its harm by obliterating brain cells. Be that as it may, it takes AD an extensive effort to demonstrate any effect, if it needs to decimate a wilderness of brain cell connections. Conversely, AD can show decently fast in the wake of invading the brain if it just needs to obliterate just a moderately couple of cellular connections, similar to an island with a single palm tree. Casual brain fitness games offer people a variety of balanced, logically based exercises wrapped inside a fun and connecting with an experience that is available to even first-time gamers. By offering incitement over the range of the brain, and sloping the difficulty such that expands the multifaceted nature of the undertakings, brain games can provide people with a successful method for increasing their brain reserve, yet still have the intrigue of casual gaming entertainment.

Adjusting and Maintaining the Brain

Although associations in the brain fitness industry sometimes use varying phrasing, and may reasonably compose brain fitness into various classifications, there is a general agreement concerning the significant areas of the brain. At Fit Brains (www.fitbrains.com), we partition our games into five noteworthy classes: Memory, Concentration, Language, Visuospatial, and Executive Functions. Notwithstanding these vital areas of the brain, every space is additionally subdivided into sub-measures that are reflected inside game exercises and progression metrics. These areas are not mainly separate; they cooperate related, as various instruments in a symphony, and can be mixed to accomplish a full proportion of brain incitement. The Fit Brains platform speaks to brain equalization and brain reserve as the Fit Brains Index (FBI) and as Brain Points. If your FBI is in the "Healthy" go or higher, that is a definite pointer that you are regularly captivating in brain fitness exercise on the site. Brain Points, then again, are a sign of your total brain fitness endeavors overall games since you previously joined the site. It is profitable for players to know that both the FBI and Brain Points benefit the most from regular, adjusted activity over the five unique subjective areas. At Fit Brains, we designed our casual brain game platform on an establishment of existing psychological training research, for example, the ACTIVE study, that keeps on rising out of the fields of personal brain research and neuroscience. A noticeable neuroscientist designs the relevant parts of the platform, Dr. Paul Nussbaum, one of the leading brain wellbeing specialists in the US, and late victor of the 2007 American Society on Aging "Gloria Cavanaugh Award" for his greatness in training and instruction in the field of maturing.

The ACTIVE study, subsidized by NIH, exhibited that grown-ups can improve brain capacities with legitimate training. The brain is most beneficial when it is active and regularly challenged. With continuous brain training, the brain performs ideally and can keep up its capacities as the years progressed. Notwithstanding brain fitness games, the other essential parts of a healthy brain way of life incorporate physical fitness, nourishment, socialization, and reflection/otherworldliness.

The Right Motivation: Brain Fitness or Entertainment

To offer the benefits of brain fitness games to the most significant potential audiences, it is essential to think about the motivations and interests of the potential socioeconomics. A few people are searching for something to enable them to exercise their brain, while others are only searching for entertainment, however, will likewise likely welcome the additional estimation of brain fitness. A compelling, mainstream brain fitness experience enables users to pick their very own motivations while furnishing them with chances to grow their points of view, and either become familiar with their brains or be urged to challenge themselves with more significant entertainment-based achievements. On the brain fitness side of the condition, Fit Brains offers a suite of devices that track a wide range of player-progression metrics over the different exercises. This incorporates a balance between every one of the significant brain areas, just as focused proposals dependent on progressively calibrated parameters identified with every one of the psychological sub-measures. To adjust the offering, there is likewise a progression of brain aerobics instructors that guide players through a reasonable brain exercise over a predetermined timeframe, extending from 3 to 30 days. For the individuals who are progressively roused by the entertainment parts of the site, there is additionally an accumulation of meta-game motivating forces designed to urge players to visit regularly and play a wide variety of brain games. These highlights incorporate Brain Points, Trophies, Achievements, Leaderboards, and Social/Community Gaming. They are each proposed to support a progressively "sticky" brain fitness experience, by welcoming players to come back to the games as often as possible and expand their skills or win fabulous prizes that go past the games themselves.

At last Casual Experience

A standout amongst the most critical objectives of brain fitness games, just as casual gaming, all in all, is to be available to the most significant variety of audiences. As the market grows and acquires more people that are new to games, this turns out to be significantly increasingly troublesome. One of the most significant challenges is to find the correct level of game difficulty that can oblige a full scope of both experienced gamers, just as those playing games for their first time. A few games offer user-picked difficulty settings that can be scary or confounding to new users, and regularly don't oblige the entire range of player capacities; different games have just a single level of difficulty progression designed to fit everybody. At Fit Brains, our casual brain-fitness games are designed to suit the way that a significant number of our site individuals are regularly new to computer games. To limit issues with "user-picked" or "one-estimate fits-all" difficulty settings, we have built up a versatile database framework that enables us to offer customized gameplay experiences through a variety of progression-diagramming and friend bunching components. This innovation allows for us to accumulate significant user metrics from different parts inside each game to set baselines that are pertinent to every user and that are stood out from actual examples got from the more extensive site user populace. This information is displayed to the end user as brain fitness metrics, which likewise incorporates brain exercise suggestions and brain training circuits. The information is additionally used to customize every user session, by adjusting every one of the games to a variety of identifiable parameters, including scoring, play time, content openness, intellectual difficulty, and that's only the tip of the iceberg. After some time, the database keeps on adjusting to every player and give by and by tuned, casual brain fitness gaming experiences for everybody. By using a self-tuning backend framework, users of any level can join the adventure and find both challenge and reward on an individual level. This attention on personalization permits the brain fitness experience to be victorious and furthermore available to the most stretched out audiences conceivable. All together for brain fitness games to resound effectively with mainstream audiences, it is essential that they give the correct harmony among science and entertainment. The science expands the game past a minor "brain topic" into a powerful device for self-awareness. The entertainment encourages people to keep up the motivation to take an interest in a healthy activity regularly. Brain fitness games may share vast numbers of similar chances and challenges found inside the casual games industry, yet the focused wellbeing center can reverberate all the more profoundly with players, which like this enables the sector to grow and attract more large audiences that might be significantly more casual than the current ones.

How to Develop Your Right Brain?
Numerous new books and procedures guarantee to develop the mental abilities of the brain. Research shows that if you exercise your less overwhelming part of the brain, the other part will likewise improve. Be that as it may, except if you exercise your feeble mental side satisfactorily, you are probably not going to be an entire brainer. There might be times when you think you used the right side of the brain, and you perhaps right. Notwithstanding, it is essential to use it every now and again, not at times. Research shows that by adulthood, 98% of the populace become left-brainer. It is in this manner, vital that we discover ways to activate the right brain, to adjust our mental abilities. There are numerous tools, techniques, and exercises to keep your right brain dynamic. Your creativity and efficiency can be amplified through explicit right-brain focused exercises. Albeit a few people have high IQ levels and are considered astute, they may need

creativity because of distressing weights on their mental or passionate energies. Left brain predominance can be a deterrent to your ability to give up and relax more, which is a right brain activity.

B-Techniques and Tools to Stimulate Your Right Brain:
Right brain actuation tools are various and incorporate different exercises, including creative writing, brain games, tests, crossword puzzles, word games, and word affiliation. In any case, the fundamental useful tools are sports, nature, mind mapping, meditation, visualization, rub, brainstorming, shading therapy, fragrance based treatment, pressure point massage, peripheral vision (hakalau), breathing techniques and hypnosis.

1-Jigsaw Puzzles: You can activate the right brain once you start to use spatial, visual, and perceptual detecting. At whatever point you collect a jigsaw puzzle and attempt to make sense of how to relate the pieces to one another, you are in effect utilizing spatial discernment. Using the parts for the last picture is accessing the visual judgment. As indicated by Michael Pitek of The Performance Group, these mental exercises are stimulant to the right brain.

2-Brainstorming: This can be a group or individual brainstorming. It was initially developed in the 1950s by Alex Osborn as a useful tool to get solutions to problems. It resembles a casual way to take care of issues in a relaxed setting, utilizing your horizontal reasoning. Research shows that individual brainstorming is more effective than the group. It is tied in with concentrating on a problem and attempting to create whatever number solutions as could be expected under the circumstances. It empowers the free progression of thoughts without analysis or assessment or judgment, with a standard time utmost of 30 minutes. By keeping away from the assessment procedure, you in effect "shut off" your left brain and enable the right side to begin thinking and working creatively.

3-Sports: Sports are excellent exercise for the body, just as incredible right brain exercises. Physical activities develop suddenness and visual imaging ability. Sports are exercises for the body and similarly crucial for the mind, particularly the right brain. Research shows that between 20-30 minutes of nonstop activity, the brain begins discharging endorphins that help support a positive state of mind and feeling great. Endorphins are released from the right brain. Consequently, the more you exercise, the higher activity happens in your right brain. Additionally, during any game, athletes need to settle on brisk choices about the development of the score of the game, and they have to access spatial as well as visual parts of the right brain to achieve those choices.

4-Peripheral Vision (Hakalau): The technique is called peripheral vision and fundamentally means extending your imagination to see into the outskirts. This is something contrary to foveal perception, the strong concentrated idea that you would have if you were, for instance, stringing a needle. You will turn out to be increasingly mindful of the development of objects instead of on shading or the objects themselves. This technique is likewise called Hakalau in the Hawaiian convention of Huna, however, has additionally been known as the Zen look, the Silent Witness, and an assortment of different terms. It is a technique of changing your sight, and at last, improving your vision. The ideal way to rehearse Hakalau is to discover a spot without any diversions, relax, and take a couple of full breaths. As you center around the edges, relax and keep your eyes open. You may feel minimal languid, which is very ordinary. Studies demonstrate that the use of peripheral vision will trigger the parasympathetic sensory system, an activity that happens at the right side of the brain. It is essential to take note of that Hakalau is additionally useful in actuating change, like hypnosis.

5-Meditation: Meditation is a standout amongst the most dominant mind tools at any point developed. Studies demonstrate that meditation improves memory, creativity, knowledge, readiness, and it synchronizes the two parts of the brain. It is realized that it will enhance the physical, mental, and emotional wellbeing. Numerous spiritualists have their understudies develop increasingly internal and mystic mindfulness through meditation. It works because it kills the steady stream of thoughts that control the more significant part of our heads. To get the best effects of meditation, it is ideal for sitting calm and inhaling gradually and focussing on body sensations.

For over 2,500 years, Buddhist priests have drilled meditation for otherworldly development. They likewise used meditation for different benefits, for example, tranquility, internal quality and to access oblivious thoughts and feelings. As indicated by Harvard Mahoney Neuroscience Letter, fall 2006, vol 12. no. 3, Harvard Medical School researchers have found that regular meditation can likewise change the structure of our brains. A group is driven by Sara Lazar, Ph.D., a neuroscientist at Massachusetts General Hospital and an educator in brain science at HMS, found that meditation expanded thickness in the locales of the brain related with consideration and preparing tactile info.

6-Visualization: Visualization is tied in with envisioning or seeing things in your mind. Creative visualization is to deliberately choose an image and see it in your account. if you need to shed pounds, you envision a picture of you being thin. Visualization is a technique used by everybody, whether they are aware of it or not. The right brain and the unconscious mind UM use the language of images. To discuss straightforwardly with your UM, use images or visualization techniques. You need to see yourself doing it in mind, and after that, you can execute it. This is the reason in sports; athletes who use visualization techniques show signs of improvement scores and accomplish higher execution level.

7-Creative Writing: Some techniques are effective in "closing off" the left brain, enabling the right side to be progressively dynamic. Creative writing courses frequently use this strategy to battle "writer's square." The consistent left side can be inert during such exercises as meditation (rehashing a mantra or word again and again) or intangible conditions. The right brain is then ready to "access" our awareness, filling our thoughts with images. One way to use creative writing is to keep a diary and write how encounters and occasions make you feel. You will write about your feelings and feelings about the situation as opposed to portraying the situation. Rather than "I got turned down for the advancement," write how you felt about it. This exercise is outlandish for some left-brainers however accommodating in activating your right brain.

8-Nature: its an undeniable fact that individuals who are connected with nature are right-brainers. Living in environment is a standout amongst the best tools for activating your right brain. Life will keep you in a steady state of Theta, a right brain state. Your feeling of anxiety will be least, yet additionally, your mental sharpness and your memory will be an ideal level. Being connected with nature empowers you to kill the diagnostic side of you and instead "feel" the encompassing condition, which is a run of the mill right brain activity.

9-Breathing Techniques: There are numerous sorts of breathing. Some breathing techniques are astounding for boosting white platelets and in this way, useful for the insusceptible framework. Hand to hand fighting breathing is generally excellent for expanding body vitality. Other breathing tools are for discharging pressure like Reichian therapy. Moderate breathing is likewise useful for accessing Theta state, and hence, can activate the right side of the brain. Blending breathing with hypnosis is useful for some benefits, and practically all are right brain-based.

10-Hypnosis: Self-hypnosis or hypnosis downloads are both extremely effective in invigorating your right brain, notwithstanding numerous different benefits. In hypnosis, under light stupor, you are in Theta state, a positive state for your brain. Under Theta, you can activate your memory capacities and discharge positive hormones like Serotonin and Endorphins. Under profound daze, you are in Delta state, the most robust state for your body and brain. In Delta, your brain speed backs off to a range between 0.1-4 cycle/second. This is where all wellbeing recovery happens. Under Delta, your body reproduces new cells. Your Unconscious Mind UM reacts to all recommendations. The change will happen all the more profoundly and rapidly under these 2 states. Theta and Delta are both right-brain exercises.

Head Games for a Better World
Bad Day? STOP. Here are how to reboot your brain.

To achieve goals in life, love, wellness, business, leadership, and to find opportunity and triumph in past knocks and wounds, I've made "Brain Games" to play on myself. They work like a "Brain Reboot" - re-setting it to capacity best. These games have turned my life around, helped me to achieve goals in life and in being an excellent rendition of myself. The games change nothing in reality and change everything in mine.

Possibly they will work for you, as well.

Attempt these straightforward systems for pivoting a - we should call it a bad day - for the present.

(1) THE LUCKY LINE GAME

DO THIS: If you think you are having a bad day, stop whatever you're accomplishing for a couple of moments. Pause to think.
Consider the LUCKY LINE: Imagine every one of the people in the world lined up from the luckiest to the unluckiest. Pause for a moment to visualize them waiting in the hopeful line. Visualize the line extending over lush slopes, crosswise over shorelines, down a tree-lined lane on a bright day. Visualize the people waiting in the Lucky Lines, moving their weight, folding their arms, scratching their heads, waiting. At that point cast your eyes initially up to the luckiest, at that point down the line to think about the people at the wrong end of the Lucky Line, people who can't sustain their youngsters, got in war zones, perhaps in Somalia where arms and legs get slashed off for someone's game, and the remainder of their lives can't scratch their very own bothersome nose. Incomprehensible, however, attempt. You are just envisioning the hatred that too many are living. Attempt to be them for a moment.
Presently, back to you. What was it that you imagined was a problem? Truly? We, as a whole, realize that getting life into viewpoint leads to appreciation, which changes everything. Be that as it may, it's not in every case be appreciative for things we've come to take as given, because we've known no other way. This "Lucky Line" strategy even helped me when I was experiencing difficulty readjusting after an ambush. I stopped by a shoreline, took a gander at the purplish-blue ocean and bright

cloudless blue sky, and felt just hurt. I quieted down to imagine the Lucky Line. It took my concentration back to the present and the magnificence around me. Before long enough as opposed to harming, my thoughts went to the way that I was fine - just my inner self was wounded for putting myself in the wrong situation, confiding in the wrong person. No doubt, life isn't reasonable. Furthermore, we should send up a little prayer of thanks that life is unjust because we are positive on the high end of the lucky line. If you can read this, you can read, have opportunity-that is fortunate. If you are reading this on an electronic gadget, if you are sheltered and very much bolstered, you are one of the lucky ones-not make any difference what else is occurring and who may have more, we are more fortunate than most.

MORE "REBOOT BRAIN GAMES":

(2) WORD EXCHANGE. Attempt to stop utilizing the word 'problem' substituting the word 'challenge rather.'
The subliminal has no comical inclination. The intuitive hears and assimilates each word you state to yourself and the world. Problems are profound. Challenges animate our purpose. Problems are "Poor me" and challenges and "I'm going to demonstrate the world!" Change the negative words you state even to yourself. The change to yourself is fantastic.

(3) ALTERNATE NARRATIVE
BACK TO THE "BAD" DAY? If you think you are having that 'bad day' we talked about prior (what will we call it now?), or you're in a situation, similar to a traffic jam, trouble paying bills, irritating collaborators; attempt these words for viewpoint. "This isn't my first decision of how to go through the day, yet if this is my most noticeably terrible problem, I'm honored." - or these words in case you're fretful in a traffic jam, someone is blocking your way in the market, stuck in the air terminal, and so on- "Waiting for this won't substantively change my life." Practice this in irrelevant situations, with the goal that you build up 'otherworldly muscle memory,' and tolerance comes all the more frequently. For instance, if someone is blocking the supermarket aisle choosing Grape Nuts and Granola, rehash to yourself how the additional 15 seconds won't

change your life. Now and again, the person will proceed onward without seeing you. If they do acknowledge, they blocked you and begin to apologize-grin and let them know not to stress to take as much time as is needed. You will watch a little, lovely, swell of kindness go from you to them.

HOW DO YOUR TINY ACTS OF KINDNESS RESONATE? We'll never honestly know, however perhaps that person blocking the aisle simply lost his employment, and possibly your moment of persistence implies he won't return home and shout at his better half, and probably the spouse won't hit the kids, and maybe the kid won't kick the feline, and perhaps the feline won't scratch your kid, and perhaps nothing returns to you so rapidly, yet everything returns. The day after my 21st birthday I went to London for 5 days and coincidentally remained 6 years (a story for another day). A few people were phenomenally kind to me. Those people, regardless, disclosed to me that when they visited the USA, Americans were extraordinarily helpful to them, and this was their method for giving back. You don't need to have confidence in God, previous existences, or karma to perceive how kindness resounds.

(4) START IN YOUR CORE: The impacts of this next idea on everyday life is stunning. This is one of the core thoughts which changed my core being. Being great doesn't begin with your activities. It starts in the core of your heart. It's insufficient for your behavior to be kind-your very thoughts about others must be kind. In what capacity will this change your life? Think about this: If someone is 90% crumby and 10% great, and you search for that 10%, you find that 10%. You set yourself in a 10% better world. More than that, if you have confidence in people, they will, for the most part, attempt to satisfy your belief-they will be better people because of your belief. Everyone wins.

BRINGING THE BEST OF "REBOOT BRAIN GAMES" for YOURSELF and THE WORLD

DON'T STOP AT FEELING BETTER-THERE IS A WHOLE LOT BETTER TO FEEL!!!

The real power in the 'Reboot Brain Games' isn't merely to use people in your creative mind to give yourself a superior day. That would resemble running a long distance race and plunking down just before the end goal.

(5) GIVE BACK: Find someone less lucky than yourself and help them.
Most significant shhhhh. Don't tell anybody what you did. Don't anticipate much appreciated. Putting your regard for honors, much appreciated, acclaim or getting your name on a divider will deny you of the excellent advantage of being and doing great. Instead, thank the person you helped for enabling you to be of administration to them. Use these ideas in help of self, and to lead those in your life. Find the gentlest opportunities to put the views on the table for others to get when they are ready. "At the point when the best leaders work is done, the people say 'we did this without anyone else's help'" (Tao). One of the improving encounters of wearing my jewelry is that when people compliment the natural magnificence, it offers a chance to open discussions, to know each other better, to lead with ideas. You don't require the jewelry. Every one of these ideas and more is in the book "Plans forever. A Step by Step Guide to Happiness," which is composed, utilizing the figurative jewelry as an outline, empowering me to share ideas at the most minimal conceivable cost for others. Each page is intended to be a jewel you can clutch for an increasingly beautiful life. If you need jewelry, it's merely usefully fantastic as a device to achieve your goals - and it's everything accessible in a wide assortment of costs by utilizing silver or gold, white sapphires, CZ or precious stones or specially made only for you.

Ten Good Habits for the Brain
I'm sure you've heard it previously: the brain resembles a muscle. So, the more you use it, the more grounded it gets. If your brain cells (neurons) aren't utilized, they will wilt and kick the bucket. Anyway, you can develop a good save and grow new pathways. What pursues are things you can do in your life that will give your brain a good workout, keep it sustained and in some instances, change your brain. These propensities will benefit you now and ideally pay off later on, as they may help anticipate dementia and Alzheimer's disease.

1 **Practice positive thinking**

At the point when awful things occur in your life, disclose to yourself that you will get past them. Realize that you have the quality and backing to do as such and they won't keep going forever. Interestingly, relish when good things come your way as you experience your day attempt and see the good on the planet and other people. By thinking like this, new pathways are framed in the brain. Indeed the brain truly can change, and it is known as neuroplasticity. By building up an uplifting mindset, your brain has indeed assembled pristine, positive pathways. How good is that?

Moreover, New York University researchers found that when people occupied with hopeful thinking, it activated the rostral front cingulate and the amygdala. These parts of the brain are both engaged with emotional responses and are likewise influenced by depression. So by getting into the idealistic propensity, your emotional reactions will be better, and you will reduce your risk of suffering from depression. The last motivation to persuade you to be idealistic is it is accepted that positive musings can discharge serotonin, a brain compound that makes you feel incredible. So you end up inclination far and away superior, on account of those unique glad musings you had.

2 Engage in standard exercise

Exercise has such a significant number of benefits to both your psychological and physical health, and research keeps on discovering an ever increasing number of purposes behind working out. The benefits to your brain are, and I have incorporated a portion of the features beneath. Ongoing speculations in advancement recommend we are more astute as a result of physical activity. Early precursors would run after their prey (perseverance running), and anthropologists suggest this prompted brain improvement in people. There is research that shows improved memory execution after participants had been running. Additionally, a 2007 Columbia University study discovered working out four times a week lead to increased neuron creation in the dentate gyrus, an area critical to memory. John Ratey has researched broadly the focal points practicing offers the brain and notes that in the short term, you will see a honing in your attention for a couple of hours after exercise. Perhaps if you battle to center at work, an excellent time to exercise would be toward the beginning of the day. In the long haul, it might avoid Alzheimer's disease. Exercise has been shown to reduce hypertension. If you have hypertension, you have an increased risk of suffering a brain drain, which may result in long haul brain damage. When you exercise, various synapses are discharged in the brain, including endorphins, serotonin, dopamine, and norepinephrine. These are naturally-occurring mood boosters, which reduce your risk of depression. Research by Weuve et al. (2004) at the Harvard School of Public Health discovered exercise reduced intellectual decrease in more established ladies. The benefits were shown for ladies in their 80s who strolled only an hour and a half a week. Be that as it may, the more dynamic the person was, the higher the benefits. Exercise is thought to increase neural strands, neurotransmitters, and vessels. Another study by Duff et al. (2008) found that more seasoned people who strolled slower did not also execute in psychological tests as people who strolled quicker. A sign of a moderate walk is somebody who took over 17 seconds to walk 50 feet. So keep up your strolling routine now for later benefits. It is apparent there are both short term and long haul gains for your brain health when you exercise. Remember to appreciate what you're doing and blend things up a bit to keep your brain alert.

3 Go dancing

When you move, there is a lot to consider. Fast choices must be made; you should focus, you should remember the moves, know about your partner, monitor your body in space, and be in contact with the beat of the music. It isn't astounding to realize then that move activates a wide range of parts of the brain - giving both your brain and body a viable workout. Your cerebral cortex and hippocampus are utilized when you are dancing, and dancing requires complex neural pathways. Through the development of these new pathways, your brain is getting bigger and more grounded and increasingly impervious to personal issues in later life. A New England Journal of Medicine report contrasted a variety of recreational exercises with see which ones reduced the risk of dementia. People who moved all the time had a 76%

reduced risk of dementia. This reduced risk was more significant than reading or doing crossword puzzles, both advantageous exercises.

4 Eat healthily and not all that much

For good physical and emotional wellness keep a regular eating regimen high in whole foods, fruit, and vegetables. Anyway, certain goods are suitable for the brain. These include fruit, vegetables, and proteins, for example, eggs, soy, beans, nuts, and seeds. Cinnamon, rosemary, turmeric, basil are altogether thought to help secure against Alzheimer's disease. Drinking fruit or vegetable juice may help secure damage to brain cells as they contain large amounts of polyphenols, which are cancer prevention agents. A 2006 University of South Florida study discovered people who drank such juices were more reluctant to build up Alzheimer's disease. Of course, a, generally speaking, healthy lifestyle may have been essential to such people, so it's not just about the juice. It additionally appears that eating an excessive amount of can prompt changes in the brain. Eating such a large number of fatty sustenances (those with lots of fat and sugar) can make the brain change, so it makes it almost certainly a person will indulge. The changes are like what happens when a person ends up dependent on medications. Another study demonstrated that overeating could increase a person's risk of memory misfortune. People more than 70 who ate somewhere in the range of 2143 and 6000 calories a day were twice as liable to be determined to have mellow subjective hindrance contrasted with the individuals who ate somewhere in the field of 600 and 1525 calories every day. The risk was not apparent for the individuals who ate under 2143 calories per day. It is estimated that overeating causes brain changes that brought about memory issues.

5 Switch off the television

Observing an excess of television can increase your risk of building up Alzheimer's as indicated by a 2005 study distributed in Brain and Cognition. The risk ascended by 1.3% for each extra hour a day spent sitting in front of the television. Not exclusively is television viewing a detached activity, yet additionally the more hours spent in front of the crate implies less time accessible for different exercises that will give your brain a good workout.

6 Play video games

On the off chance that you should sit in front of the television, you should be dynamic while you are there. The appropriate response, in all honesty, is video games. With some restraint, of course. Researchers are finding that playing video games is doing the brain properly. Bavelier's research has shown gamers are more engaged than non-gamers and are capable of tracking data. Brain outputs demonstrated gamers' minds were progressively effective and faster when it came to focusing (they can track 6 things immediately. The standard is 4). Other research has shown gamers to be progressively innovative, better leaders, have predominant perceptual aptitudes and improved deftness. Presently as a COD widow, do I tell my better half this?

7 Puzzles and games

Puzzles and games activate various parts of the brain contingent upon the sort. Participate in anything that makes you think. Play chess, rationale puzzles, re-arranged words, strategy games, crosswords, Sudoku, Mahjong, jigsaws, card games, scrabble. Attempt to complete a variety to exercise various areas of your brain and increase the multifaceted nature once they get excessively straightforward.

Bunge and Mackey had students play board, card, and video games that tested either their processing speed or reasoning ability. Following 8 weeks, the reasoning ability prepared students saw a 32% increase in their non-verbal insight scores. The processing speed made students saw their speed scores increase by 27%.

8 Learn new things

When you discover some new information, you create new connections among neurons and existing ones get more grounded. Learning new things isn't just about taking courses or extending your insight into new areas. It's tied in with adjusting to changes that happen each day. For example, at whatever point your preferred programming or web-based life application gets a redesign, you may gripe about the change. Notwithstanding, consider your brain for a minute. It's utilized to the old way of working and doesn't need to work exceptionally difficult to operate the product. The change implies you have to reconsider, which prompts the formation of new pathways effectively. You've given your brain a workout. Along these lines, whenever you experience a test, instead of giving up, resolve to ace it. Not exclusively will you feel a feeling of accomplishment; however, your brain will be more significant as well!

9 Don't consider knowledge to be a fixed thing

Research by Dweck and associates demonstrated that when students were instructed to perceive that the brain shapes new connections and develops through learning, the gathering saw an increase in their math grades. As grown-ups, it's easy to accept that we as a whole are learning and improvement is finished. At this point, you are either good at something, or you are most certainly not. I trust this book has shown that your brain can proceed to develop and that pathways should you have as much as possible. Shake off any names given to you as a tyke. Give things a go, resolve to become familiar with other expertise, or face your Achilles heel. If you've chosen to work on your Achilles heel, remember that if you are battling, there is more than one way to pick up something. Give yourself another pathway to pursue.

10 Read a book

There's a lot included when you settle down to the loosening up activity of reading. Your brain is kept occupied as you have to store data about what you have read and had the option to recover it as you advance through the book. Who was that character referenced 100 pages back? You additionally activate your innovativeness and creative mind as you breathe life into the characters depicted in words in your account. This is simply fiction. There's likewise the likelihood of learning about new areas that you know nothing about by perusing the true to life segment. If you are an authority of free, encourage books, ensure you put aside time to read them.

Creativity - Calisthenics For The Brain
When all that was rushing about and working comes to an end

upon retirement age... at that point what? Question: What do I do with this extra time? "The happiest people are those that are too busy to even think about noticing whether they are or not." William Feather

* Senator Pete Domenici, from the territory of New Mexico (where I live), will retire from the Senate in 2008, following 35 years in the Congress. He was diagnosed with an incurable brain disease, which changes a person's personality. (See: Welcome to the Funny Farm/mental health)

* The unthinkable occasions at Virginia Tech in 2007, has shown every one of us that we would do well to pay attention to mental health and all work together to eliminate the stigma associated with mental illness. None of us are getting any more youthful.

* I thought nothing about dementia until I was in the hospital in 2005. One of the different veterans had dementia, and the medical caretaker told me that he was 48 years old, with a mind of a three-year-old. How terrible! Some people have genuinely been dealt a lousy hand in life! (See: Remembering Manuel...)

When I crossed over the 40 and 50-year-old in age...it didn't bother me. Be that as it may, when I crossed over the 60-year-old mark...it bothered me. To use a football analogy...I'm now entering the fourth quarter of my life, and I am quickly approaching the two-minute warning, and so on. Like it or not, the clock is ticking down for us all.

We all need to remain in shape, both physically and mentally. Not being a psychologist, how does a person stay in shape mentally? By staying active, and there are many spots to visit on the Internet that can help, and there are only a couple.

From: Design For Strong Minds.com

Research has shown that like different muscles, brain function is used it...or lose it proposition. The more aging adults challenge and use their minds, the more agile their brains remain.

From: Eldr.com

Brain exercises can enable you to keep sharp and help avoid dementia. Your brain is amazing! It just weighs around three pounds and is small enough to hold in your hands, and yet it contains more than 100 billion nerve cells that orchestrate every part of your considerations, your perceptions, and your behavior.

If you deal with your brain, like different organs and muscles, it will remain stable and vibrant.

From: My Brain Trainer.com
Contains short, fun, individual exercises designed to stimulate different pieces of your brain. Similarly, as ordinary work-outs in a gym, improve your physical fitness, a standard mental work-out improves your cognitive function and brain processing speed.

Mainstream brain exercises include:
* Cross-word puzzles; I admire people who can do crossword puzzles because they have a large vocabulary. I'm not a fanatic of crossword problems, because my vocabulary is around 14 words...and that is up from 13 words in 1968. Let me see...I need a three letter word for a four-legged animal that barks...m-mmm-let me think about it...
* Ordinary puzzles; In 2005, I was in the hospital for more than a quarter of a year, and there were different patients in the ward, that worked on those problematic, gigantic puzzles with more than 1,000 pieces. I don't have the patience to do this. However, a can appreciate the people who worked on these puzzles.
* Rubik's solid shape; This type of puzzle stimulates the brain all right...right into a mental institution! These type of problems are suited for a seven-year-old, who can do them quickly, and not for us older adults. (who are you calling old?) I experience difficulty connecting the dots or painting by the numbers, so what am I going to do with one of these puzzles?
For me, creativity is the response to keep my mind busy and to get the needed calisthenics. I've always considered myself as a trustworthy idea person...both good and bad ideas. We don't have any desire to discuss the stinkers. I've still considered myself a standout amongst the most intelligent people In the world, and It just fitted that I show you my credentials.

- Credentials: Jerry Aragon, BS; MS; Ph.D; MD; KFC; T.G.I.F; BMW; CBS; TLC; CCR; GMA; ETC; ETC; ETC

- Business card: (silly card) I have used my stupid card for around seven years now, and it contains the standard contact information in addition to the following; Jerry Aragon; The Humor Doctor M.D. (Mentally Disturbed) Specializing in mal-practice; House call

- Wood carving: As a woodcarver for more than 25 years, I've carved more than 200 original figures in wood, and all have taken patience; coordination; and concentration. I've sold almost everything I've made at expressions and specialties shows, galleries, and gift shops. I've always loved the test of creating something that has never been done. A couple of my pieces include; Parents Running Away From Home; Flu Bug...sick in bed with the flu; a little wild bear fledgling sitting in a red and white high chair; a VW with two front ends; a lion sitting in a bathtub and so forth. For more than 25 years, this is one way I have kept my mind busy and stimulated.
"Anybody can make the simple complicated. However, creativity makes the complicated simple." Charles Mingus
Creativity is not an 8 to 5 job. For many of us, creativity is all day, every day and the mind works all the time...even while we're sleeping. Some of the best ideas I have gotten, have come while I was snoozing, and after I wake, I need to write them down quickly before they escape!
- Writing: Writing is therapeutic for me. Some hobbies are expensive, however with writing all you need is a pencil, pad and make sure to bring your ideas and imagination. Printing should be possible pretty much anyplace. In 2005, I was in the hospital for more than three months...and heck...I composed more than 100 pages for my book, and so forth.

CHAPTER SEVEN

Super Foods For Arthritis and Meditations to Help With Arthritis

FROM SUPER FIT TO SUDDEN CHRONIC ILLNESS

One day I was an incredibly fit individual, practicing yoga and meditation daily; the following day, I arose in chronic pain. Rapidly limb by limb over the coming days and weeks, I step by step turned out to be increasingly disabled. A couple of months after the fact I was told devastating news that I had a disabling condition called spondyloarthritis. How did this occur so all of a sudden with no sign of manifestations previously? I was stunned, bewildered, and frightened as the consultants revealed to me how serious it was and how it would probably be with me for the remainder of my life. My condition was terrible to the point that I could scarcely walk and even from a pessimistic standpoint I must be pushed in a wheelchair which made me cry since I couldn't see how I had got to such a spot so rapidly having dependably been fit and healthy. I was in a lousy place, rationally and physically. I couldn't concentrate on meditation, especially when the medication brought me into its inhumane chemical trances; needless to state the side effects over that were challenging most definitely. One of the drugs I needed to take completely hindered my mind from creativity, which was devastating for me as I write and record meditations.

Without any weaning period, CHRONIC Anemia AND DEPRESSION WERE MY COMPANIONS

My nature being extremely positive I embarked on fighting Arthritis with food. My remedies I believed in so truly were not working, so I enabled my Consultants to medicate me, as the pain was intense to the point that it was a close impossible to rest for the more significant part an hour at a time. I felt crushed as my Consultant disclosed to me I would need to grapple with the diagnosis, so reluctantly I said yes to steroids, which made my condition more awful. The following course of treatment was nonsteroid arthritis anti-inflammatory medications, which offered some relief from my chronic pain and enabled me to function in an increasingly worthy manner. I experienced some relief. Be that as it may, throughout the months I wasn't getting any better, the inflammation never went down, and I was beginning to spiral in and out of mini-depressions with the constant pain. I looked so pale as I currently had chronic anemia. My Consultant suddenly accepting me off my medication as he associated the pill was the reason with my anemia. I was left without any weaning period, and the leading pain killers permitted were paracetamol which didn't do much or tramadol that thumped me out, needless to state I was feeling exceptionally discouraged by this stage. During the time I never surrendered and was continually trying new remedies, juicing, homemade foods, the arthritis diet, cider vinegar, dark tie molasses, natural medications, homeopathic, alternative therapies, pain machines. I practically exhausted all my options. I was frantic to walk again with straightforwardness. I so wanted to tend my garden which I adored and had so severely dismissed, as I was unfit to twist down. Indeed my memory humors me now as I think back to how bad I was even under the least favorable conditions; my felines used to get extremely impatient with their suspended food dish in the air that was coming down millimeter by millimeter, which appeared to take an eternity to reach the ground. They would jump up trying to assist in pulling it to the cold earth and sometimes did with a mighty accident spilling food everywhere throughout the floor!

A MIRACLE - I DISCOVERED SUPER FOODS FOR ARTHRITIS
I read books, tried everything I knew about that could help, spent large measures of cash until I felt I had exhausted every one of my options, and felt empty. Nothing helped. I exercised daily; however, it was misery. One day I was surfing the net once more in the hope I had missed something, and by chance, I ran over a case cast about cocoa beans by David Wolfe. I couldn't believe the potential of superfoods for Arthritis and the health-enhancing properties cocoa contained. I felt excited and optimistic. So started the following period of my journey of consuming cocoa daily, one of the beneficial superfoods for people living with Arthritis. I felt hope again without precedent for months. Cocoa diverted my life around literally from the day I was first accepting it as within hours I felt my mood change because of the typical mood enhancing chemicals it contains and within days my pain

was less, and my inflammation diminished. This crunchy bean that was progressively like a nut with bitter chocolate enhance made me feel great without precedent for a long time. I noticed my walking was improving, and my energy levels were the best they had been for a long time, which was terrific. I felt cheerful again. I was impressed to the point that I wanted to become familiar with superfoods for Arthritis. I went over recommendations to take cocoa nibs along with goji berries for a progressively intense health remedy and the complimentary taste.

HEALTH BENEFITS OF COCOA AND GOJI BERRIES

Goji berries are referred to as the upbeat berry as they are accounted for to have mood lifting properties just as many other desirable health benefits. The combination of Cocoa and Goji berries from my experience are incredibly ground-breaking. Cocoa is a standout amongst the most nutrient rich and complex foods known to man and individual specialists, is considered to be the leading antioxidant food and is the best wellsprings of magnesium of any known food, which many people living with Arthritis are deficient. It is additionally a rich wellspring of iron, which helped with my anemia. Various benefits that grabbed my eye from my examination were as per the following:

Goes about as an anti-depressant and balances the mood; Balances the brain chemistry; Builds solid bones; Detoxifies the liver; Helps with healthy pancreas functioning; Balances blood sugar; Builds a stress resistance shield; Regulates inflammatory and immune reactions in blood vessel walls; Contains anandamide "The Bliss Chemical", serotonin and endorphins; Cocoa beans/cacao is a standout amongst the most nutrient rich and complex foods known to man. I can't express firmly enough how these two gifts of nature have helped to turn my life around. I managed to fall off all painkillers within seven days of taking cocoa and have been free from any medication for a long time now. One year after my diagnosis, I have solidarity to walk and climb steps. I can tend my garden with joy and happiness. I have consistent energy and now have shading back in my cheeks. The most important thing is that I presently have a steady clear mind and strength as I have never experienced. It's such a joy to have my very own authentic account back, clear of chemical blockages, which has enabled me to be true to my inner self again. For quite a long time I couldn't meditate, as my mind was affected by chemicals from medication which places me into a chemical haze, far from mindfulness. Presently I am on the way of wellbeing; meditation is a big piece of my daily life again. It has helped to clear my mind of all the injury of the trail of painful energy illness abandoned. For quite a long time, the chemicals I was consuming daily appeared to remove me on a journey from my true self and into a somber descending spiral of eternal suffering. Superfoods for Arthritis helped me to find my way back home and re-ignited my passion for practicing meditation daily. My yoga developments are coming along nicely again, as well.

Learning IS A BLESSING - SHARING IS CARING
I hope that by sharing my experience, I may help other people. I realize we are altogether made differently as human beings, and while medication may suit a few people, it may not adapt to others. Superfoods for Arthritis might be a savior to a portion of my perusers like they were and still are to me today. Regardless of whether I reach out and help a couple of people by sharing my journey and my learning's, then I will be upbeat. As a therapist, I have practiced continuously as I preach, yet the intrusion of Arthritis into my life has since lead me to progressively more profound significant dimensions of my practice which I live and breath daily. If it's not too much trouble care for your body and your mind - they are precious - treasure them or more all please make an effort to remain true to yourself, my dear peruser.

Seven Foods to Avoid for Brain Fog Relief
"The intelligent man ought to consider that wellbeing is the best of personal favors. Give food a chance to be your medicine." - Hippocrates
It's essential to comprehend that foods reflect how we feel, and this is especially true for the individuals who battle with brain fog (depersonalization) and other anxiety reactions. A few foods fuel the framework and help maintain stable serotonin and blood sugar levels. This prompts a sharp feeling of prosperity. Different foods do the exact inverse and regularly trigger anxiety, panic attacks, feelings of brain fog, and even phobic reactions. This is the

reason it is critical to learn which foods will work for you and which foods to avoid if you endure anxiety reactions.

Foods to Avoid:

1. Sugar: Sugar will incidentally induce beautiful sensations in the brain and body however inside a brief timeframe these feelings will subside and crash, leaving the distinct impression foggy, on edge, bad-tempered, eager and lazy. Anyone who has ever battled with anxiety or brain fog will notice that sugar is their main adversary. It will likewise disturb rest designs and exacerbate feelings of OCD and Panic Attacks. Surrendering the excess use of sugar furnishes one with such dramatic alleviation that this in itself demonstrates out the fact that sugar is detrimental to anyone enduring with feelings of brain fog and anxiety. Keep in mind that chemical sugar substitutes are similarly as damaging.

2. Alcohol: Alcohol is referred to as numerous as "fluid sugar" since it is rated the highest number on the glycemic index. It will incidentally lift one's spirits, yet a precarious price is paid for this transient fantasy. Alcohol likewise affects one's blood sugar levels, feeling of prosperity, serotonin levels and results in feelings of extraordinary brain fog, anxiety, rest intrusion, fractiousness and failure to maintain stable blood sugar levels the day in the wake of soaking up. One regularly experiences spikes and drops in blood sugar levels the following day as the body attempts to reestablish stable blood sugar levels. This produces discomfort and enhanced brain fog alongside plenty of anxiety symptoms for anyone who has experienced this effect.

3. Caffeine: Unfortunately, caffeine, found in a vast number of substances, is a complicated chemical to suffer if one is touchy to brain fog and anxiety reactions. It accelerates digestion, increases heart rate, creates peevishness, enhances anxiety reactions, and is found in many foods we regularly eat. Indeed, we, as a whole, realize that coffee and tea contain caffeine and substituting these drinks with decaffeinated forms is essential, yet some decaffeinated brands still have a level of caffeine inside. Individual coffee shops that offer decaffeinated substitutes have had their decaf tried some still rate high on the caffeine chart. Your best verification is how you feel in the wake of utilizing these brands. Trust me; your body will alarm you. Likewise, natural teas, generally are without caffeine, yet there are numerous that are most certainly not. Check out your green teas and ensure you are selecting the ones that are decaffeinated since even little doses of caffeine will affect a sharpener body. Chocolates additionally carry a caffeine load, some more than others. Avoid dark chocolates as they are higher in caffeine.

4. Certain Food Additives: Sorbitol, Xylitol, Mannitol are chemicals used to improve foods and products we regularly use consistently. They are in drinks, treats, cereals, mouthwash, and toothpaste. They not just create issues with brain fog and anxiety yet additionally resentful the stomach and add to IBS symptoms too, regardless of whether you've never experienced IBS previously. They are best avoided because they have zero benefits to those with brain fog or anxiety.

5. Low-Fat Products: Whenever you see "Low Fat" on labels, you will realize the fat has been replaced with SUGAR. This is effectively recognized by perusing the names of all low-fat foods. Try not to be tricked by "low fat" claims because the sugar which replaces the fat will work superbly of adding fat to the body and at times more so than the first fat.

6. Healthy Juices: Juices are delicious and frequently give large amounts of Vitamins, essential for good wellbeing, especially Vitamin C. This is for what reason I'm not expressing to avoid juices out and out but rather instead proposing to add water to your 100% breakfast juice and by doing as such will avoid the enormous sugar rush connected with this product. You will, in any case, receive the rewards of the juice without the side effects of an excess of sugar.

7. Healthy Snacks: Read labels carefully. The more significant part of these "healthy snacks contain unmistakably more sugar and chemical products than you need to ingest. For quite a long time, people were eating products such as low-fat granola bars and rice cakes, accepting they would maintain a decent figure and feel healthy too. Not true. Their blood sugar levels took off, thus did their feelings of brain fog and manic episodes.

There are such a significant number of "clean" foods that one can get, which help maintain a healthy personality and body. Likewise, learning how to use proteins to produce balanced and stable blood sugar levels is essential. One is ready to choose how they wish to feel once they learn the basics of good eating, especially for feelings of brain fog and the anxiety condition. Shop shrewd by controlling your cart to the fringe of the market. This is the place all the fresh foods are placed. Avoid those center aisles loaded up with processed and refined foods.

Eating correctly, in conjunction with learning how to think correctly, will allow you the benefit of wiping out all impressions of brain fog and anxiety reactions.

How To Improve Your Memory
Too frequently when I pose the inquiry: "Do you have a bad memory? The automatic answer I get is an emphatic Yes!

My next question to them is to imagine a scenario in which somebody was to obtain from the state a million dollars would they overlook the person. Furthermore, this time they give me a resounding No! Not! When I ask them for what good reason that is so and they state "well it's obvious isn't it? I mean in what capacity can you possibly overlook that? So back to the original question: "for what reason do you think you have a bad memory?" This time they give me another excuse. Except if you've been diagnosed with some brain debilitating disease, there is no such thing as a bad memory. So far as that is concerned, there is no such thing as a decent memory either. What the more significant part of us have is a new mind that can be supported to develop a razor-sharp memory. The main reason why a few of us feel that we can't achieve this is they are expecting it to happen overnight and they trust that there is some pill that they can swallow that will boost their memory power. Albeit a few kinds of sustenance can here and there keep our memory power intact, what it truly boils down to is to train our brain to remember what we need and recall them when we need to. In an ongoing seminar that I conveyed; I had an 80-year-old respectable man who in the wake of having been educated on the best way to remember had the option to recall a not insignificant list of words in a brief period. This is indeed a demonstration of the way that seniority does not devastate our ability to remember. Consider this representation: what occurs if you never use a knife for an extended period? The answer is obvious - it will not be as sharp as it ought to be. However, when you've sharpened it and use it regularly, you find that it remains sharp. After some time, you find that it gets gruff again and you have to grind it afresh. This is the way your memory works. You have to sharpen your memory now and again. Much the same as you keep your physical body sound by engaging in regular exercise, you can keep your memory razor sharp by doing the following things.

Improve your power of observation
One of the key reasons why a significant number of us feel that we have a lousy memory is because we don't boost our power of observation. If you drive, how frequently have you parked your car in a multi-story carpark and were unfit to find where you've parked the car when you return? The reason why you have this issue is that when you parked your car, you failed to interface or link your vehicle to the surrounding environment. You perceive the world that is before you and your vehicle. What you need to do is to turn and have a decent take a gander at your car and see where you've parked it. Link your car to a pillar or remember the lot number where you've parked. When you are introduced to another person, the first thing that you do is to find out the person's name. But then a couple of moments later you can't remember the name. Again this is because of your absence of a power of observation. What you can do is to request that the person rehash their name if you did not get it the first time. If the person gives you a name card, take a gander at the card and make an association of the person with the name and his/her organization.

Precedent: Let say you were introduced to Theresa Lim, who is an HR manager with Alphabet Pte Ltd. Maybe you could see a "Tree" with lots of letters from the alphabets hanging from it. At that point, you know who the person is as 'tree' sounds near Theresa, and the notes on the tree may trigger your brain to recall the name of the organization she is working. However, I need to caution you here to be sensitive to this as it might look impressive on your part if you can recall the person you met, yet you certainly won't have any desire to tell the person how you remember her.

Boost your concentration

This is important if you genuinely need to develop a razor-sharp memory. You don't have to sweat over it. You could do it gradually and steadily. Boosting your concentration encourages your brain to intensify its various activities and in this way causes you to recall information with ease. You can increase your strength by trying to link a random list of words by creating a story between them. Attempt to remember an entire tune lyric by hard and sing it. You can likewise take a passage from a book or a list of countries and see whether you could remember them by hand. When you compel yourself to remember such list of items, there is a propensity for your brain to make numerous neural connections that enables you to boost your concentration and this, in turn, causes you to increase your ability to recall information with ease.

Learn another thing every day

This is a standout amongst the best ways to keep your memory razor sharp. When you learn something new every day, you will find yourself becoming increasingly progressively alert and focus on what you are doing. One effective way to do this is to learn another word from the dictionary every day and attempt to use it in your daily conversation or writing. Or on the other hand, you could keep an encyclopedia by your bedside and learn another bit of information before you rest. The Internet has many useful search engines that give you immediate access to practically any information that you need. Do whatever it takes not to search for things that you as of now have prior knowledge in. Learn something new as in that way your brain will pay heed. When you do this regularly, you will find that the further information appears to pull in your interest and this will inspire your brain to make powerful connections with existing information you have to enable you to boost your memory and make it razor sharp.

The Brain-Gut Connection

Have you at any point asked why individuals get butterflies in the stomach before a job interview or enormous execution? Or on the other hand, even why individuals upchuck at the idea of something terrible or while under severe pressure?

The reason for these essential encounters is that your digestive tract and stomach acts explicitly as a moment brain. The human digestive tract contains more than one million nerve cells... this is about a similar amount of nerves found in the spinal cord! There are more never cells in your digestive system than there is in the whole fringe nervous system. Your digestive brain and the brain in your skull are linked together using the vagus nerve. The vagus nerve "meanders" from the brain stem through the organs in the neck and thorax lastly ends in the stomach area. This has been named the "brain-gut" connection by Jordan Rubin, creator of The Makers Diet.

This second 'abdominal brain' s similarly as significant as your 'skull brain.' As per Dr. Michael Gershon, educator of life structures and cell biology at Columbia Presbyterian Medical Center in New York City depicts the body's second nervous system in his book The Second Brain:

"The brain isn't the main spot in the body that is brimming with neurotransmitters. A hundred million neurotransmitters line the length of the gut, roughly a similar number that is found in the brain... The brain in the inside must work right, or nobody will have the privilege to think by any stretch of the imagination."

Your stomach truly thinks and, can feel and express your emotions.

Brilliant Core

As per Paul Chek in Scientific Core Conditioning, the rectus abdominis is segmentally innervated by various 8 nerves. He keeps on attesting that due to the abundance of nerves that innervate the core/abdominal musculature, it capacities as though it has 8 brains.

(2) The reason for the abundance of nerve endings in the

abdominal musculature is self-evident... all through our advancement, the hardships of formative condition directed that the abdominal musculature need to be incredibly reliable just as canny. It is the abdominal musculature that is in charge of: the balancing out impact for the statement of limb movement, expanding intra-abdominal pressure to aid constrained articulation, flexion, revolution, ipsilateral isometric contraction when animated singularly, moved strain to make spinal stability by means of that thoracic-lumbar fascia (TCF), and so on. Thus, my point is clear... your abs have a lot of jobs, so they've been given a lot of brains.

Abdominal Inhibition due to emotional disturbance To emphasize... First, your digestive system acts as a moment brain and contains an equal amount of nerve cells from the spinal cord. Additionally, due to the abundance of neurotransmitters present in the stomach, it has been watched, both clinically and experientially, that it is exceedingly influenced by the emotions that we produce.

Next, it has been set up that the core musculature has "8 brains". The muscles of the abdominal are exceptionally advanced to withstand "basic man's" need to endure and flourish informative condition using useful movement designs famous for chasing just as building shelter.

Both the digestive system and the abdominal musculature are linked using the nervous system. One of the essential control centers of the nervous system, the brain, can represent the moment of truth your endeavors to smooth your abs and fabricate a stone muscular physique... and I am demonstrating how. Inside organs obtain their pain-sensitive nerve fibers from the muscular system. This implies when an organ feels pain, the brain can't decide whether it's the muscle or the organ that harms. The brain realizes which fragment of the spine that the pain message originated from. Along these lines, the brain at that point makes an impression on that specific region of the spine and tells the majority of the muscles, tissue, and organs in that region to act as though they were in pain. (

3) When you are distressed, due to emotional disturbance from - budgetary uncertainty, connections, a job that you despise or

going through an hour on the telephone with your discouraged moderately aged auntie... your stomach or second brain reacts. A portion of the particular watched reactions by this organ to emotional pain incorporates diminished or expanded blood flow, "clenching," and digestive hindrance. While this is happening, your abdominal musculature has quite recently gotten a similar message that the stomach has - "there is a pain, and we should react." Your abdominal muscles, presently seeing pain, become restrained, and lose the capacity to contact to their fullest capacity. This is valid specifically for the Transversus Abdominis, the muscle that activates the thoracic-lumbar fascia for low back stability and acts to keep your stomach "attracted." (I've quite recently demonstrated to you how mental/emotional distress causes low back pain also.)

Things being what they are, I don't get this' meaning for me?
The point that I might want to clarify is that as a comprehensive substance, your whole physiology is linked through control systems, including the nervous system. You currently comprehend why mental/emotional stability is fundamental for reliable quality and durability... particularly as it identifies with your abdominal. If you have been attempting, ineffectively, to improve your feel through incalculable crunching sessions and dieting - I welcome you to think about what you have been absent as much as half of your chance to have better wellbeing and distinct quality. Disregarding or working against your body doesn't work! What's more, you will look as high outwardly as you feel within.

What would I be able to do?
To start with, perceive that you are a coordinated system of systems and that one piece of your mind-body can't encounter injury without it influencing a few others.

Can Brain Techniques Give You the Winning Edge?
Do we concur that you and I are doubters and need a lot of proof before we accept - anything? Experience has instructed us to put stock in Cause-And-Effect, right? In any case, does science (neuroscience, really brain science) guarantee to have every one of the responses to how humans think and act? Not yet.

102

Would it be a good idea for us to keep a receptive outlook on brain techniques that future research may demonstrate to be relevant?
Example: to be at your most honed, utilizing the vast majority of your mind, raise your VIBRATIONS. What are vibrations, and how would you build them?

We, as a whole, have brain vibrations 24/7 that change our attitude, perspective, and decision-making power. The proof returned to 1924 when an Austrian therapist named Hans Berger made (created) the EEG (Electroencephalogram). It was the ultimate proof that humans are at the center - electrical systems. Our brain keeps running on electrical vibrations dependent on our activity. Example: when we are wakeful the EEG records Beta cycles every second (13 to 40 Hertz). This Beta works when our eyes are open, and we are alert and thinking. It is human consciousness. Second is Alpha brainwave cycles delivering 8-13 cycles (Hertz) every second. When we are loose, quickly alert, and close our eyes and dream, we promptly enter Alpha. Reflection is 90% in Alpha. Third, are Theta brain vibrations delivering 4-7 cycles for each second. We go into more profound relaxation, which makes inventiveness, intuition, imagination, and motivation. Incredible developments, new ideas come during Theta. Fourth is Delta brainwave vibrations, 1/2 - 4 cycles for every second. It switches on during rest and later in imagining. Consciousness rests, and Non-Consciousness dominates. After ten years in 1934, his EEG was considered "the most astonishing, wonderful and groundbreaking improvement ever of nervous system science." Now, right around 80 years after the fact scientists still use Berger's EEG for brain research. Today even eighth graders know there are four distinct sorts of electrical activity in the human brain: every ha distinctive wave examples, rhythms, and capacities. Power makes us human.

What of it
Peruse this cautiously, or you will miss its centrality. You can without much of a stretch raise your vibrations from slow-to-quick and improve your decision-making powers, investigation and intuition. Intuition and motivations are hunches and gut-reactions

that originate from our Non-Consciousness. What exactly is non-consciousness?

It couldn't be any more obvious; there are six (6) brain structures working when we are wakeful and alert. Just one of them makes us mindful of its reality - Consciousness (Beta). The other 5/6th (83.33%) of our thinking-brain are on auto-pilot. Huh? Your heart is pulsating, circulatory strain, body temperature, and safe system work naturally (auto-pilot). Pause - Consciousness has a transfer speed (capacity) of only 16 to 40 Bits of Information Per Second. Not a lot, right? Non-Consciousness (5/6th) has an ability of 11-MILLION Bits of Information. What a correlation. Our primary responsibility is to use the transfer speed (capacity) of our Non-Consciousness to attract wellbeing, better recuperating, riches, security from risk, and better associations with brain techniques. Huh?

Club

Suppose that you are at the Bellagio gambling club in Vegas. You are there to attempt to capture the Poker Tournaments. You realize how to play a not too bad hand of poker and perhaps win a jackpot or two. If you can control your attitude, your psychological state, and not be an enthusiastic better, you improve the odds in your favor.

How

Get this: many effective decisions are NOT founded on logic and reasoning. They are neuroscience dependent on your musings and feelings. The research shows - how you control your mind, brainwaves, and Rhythm will improve the odds in your favor. There are simple infant techniques to slow down your Rhythm (vibrational frequency) and develop your consideration and concentration for better decision-making.

Rhythm Technique

Plunking down, accelerate your vibrations by flagging your brain by pounding both your hands on your knees - quickly. Tap a fast rhythm for 15-30 seconds and unwind. At regular intervals do an additional 15-second arrangement of tapping. You are raising your brain vibrations. That is simple, right? Remain with me, the second component in raising your brain Rhythm (vibrational technique) is utilizing your imagination (mental perception) to make a psychological guide to achieve your goals. How? Imagine as you tap your speedy Rhythm, the cards being played out at the table. See yourself making the most brilliant decisions, and winning the jackpot. Huh? See the procedure of you taking in the jackpot. Insane? Ask Tiger Woods or other expert competitors how they rationally practice their abilities. Mental practice engraved your goal, similarly as physical exercise does. They imagine, picture and rationally observe the exact advances they will take to win (score) in tennis, baseball, and golf. They make a psychological guide on how to play, and it is changing the odds of winning. The tapping makes a focused ATTENTION and concentration, while your mind-motion pictures use Memory Neurons to trigger your winning techniques. This technique is called POLARITY, meaning approaching and active. You can use your Will Power to raise your vibrational frequency (brainwaves) to improve your odds. A few scientists accept your brainwave rhythms can attract what you center your mind around. Would you be able to imagine remaining in the progression of winning jackpots? Quit dissecting the logic and reasoning, and complete a mind-try. Attract your goals.

Sounds Dumb
"We humans can imagine something in our mind (brain). We use our Primary Visual Cortex, a similar brain structure we use to see our condition and have experienced. Humans can imagine things that don't exist, and after that, go out and make these ideas. Examples: a hand hatchet, a woodwind, the web, and one year from now's Cadillac. We recombine bits of information from our experiences and learning into NOVEL structures. The varieties are limitless." John Hoffecker. College of Colorado, Archeologist. Do you state you put stock in cause-and-impact? Complete a "mind analysis" and figure out how to win.

New Technique to Attract Success
There are two sorts of smiles, showing our TEETH alone, or consolidating showing our teeth with having crow's feet at our EYES. Have you at any point seen a display commercial of representatives (not actors) who are grinning exclusively with their

teeth? It is called PanAm grinning, and they are driving themselves to smile. A real smile is known as a Duchenne Smile, after a French nervous system specialist, and joins showing our teeth and squinting our eyes. Grinning triggers our Zygomatic Major muscle used in outward appearances. Real grinning uses your RISORIUS muscle to draw out the muscles of your mouth. At long last, your Orbitocularis Oculi, muscle makes your Eyelids squint and delivers crow's feet at your eyes.

What of it
Would you be able to make a phony smile on your face right this second?
Go on the defensive in a broad smile, and you are there. When you maintain this pretend smile
(PanAm smile) For 1-2 minutes, it turns into a real (authentic) smile (teeth and eyes). When you have a smile on your face, REAL-Or-PHONY, you trigger your brain to feel upbeat and attract positive experiences. How? You raise your vibrational frequency - it's electrical brainwaves at work.
You can't have a phony-smile on your puss and believe and act contrarily. Attempt it now.
How does this act of Will Power help us?
The act of fake grinning, acting as though you are glad because you decide to, influences your nervous system. Your brain changes from Sympathetic to your Parasympathetic Nervous System. Tune in up - your Sympathetic Nervous system contains your Fight-or-Flight reflex, (adrenaline) while your Parasympathetic causes relaxation (acetylcholine) delivers better decisions and intuitions.
At the point when your brain is energized by adrenaline, it doesn't think unmistakably or uses sound judgment. To attract your passionate longings, you need profound relaxation, which is your Parasympathetic Nervous System and the synapse - acetylcholine. It even improves your eyes by enhancing your fringe vision. So Maintain a phony smile on your face until it turns into a genuine Duchenne smile. It requires 1-2 minutes. The advantages are the arrival of stress, nervousness and dread, and the ability to settle on winning decisions throughout your life. Play the job of a grinning, cheerful individual, (stay-in-character) and your mind-body association will repeat another, better mental attitude. A few

understudies swear you become a Money-Magnet

Although it is mainly older people that are concerned with brain exercises, new research recommends that we should give more consideration to brain health from an early age.
One of every ten people beyond 65 years old have dementia. After the age of 85 it is one out of three. One research researcher has likened it to superannuation, in however much as you should begin putting resources into the health of your brain as right on time as could reasonably be expected. The decline in brain function can take decades meaning that lifestyle in the early years will impact on the brain as we age. Brain exercises are presently considered impeccably normal. It seems that wherever you go nowadays, you will come crosswise over people doing crosswords, Sudoku and different types of activities to keep the brain fit as a fiddle however in the not so distant past the idea that the brain needed exercising would have met with derision or skepticism. My husband Chris and I have dependably believed in all-encompassing health and, harking back to the eighties, we were becoming interested in another form of eye exercise. When we mentioned it among a gathering of friends and family, they thought we had lost the plot. One can imagine the thing they would have said about brain exercises. While clearly, most people need to keep everything in good working order for whatever length of time that conceivable, its a well-known fact that, dread of dementia as we age is a driving power behind the brain exercise explosion. Baby boomers, of which I am one, expect to live for a long time and they plan to accomplish more than their parents and grandparents. People need to be fit and healthy to appreciate the latter part of their lives, so brain health is becoming an accepted part of our health and wellness regime. A healthy lifestyle can possibly prevent a third of all dementia. Indeed, even people in the beginning times of the disease can, at present, make a difference if they make changes gainful to the health of their brain. Although it isn't using all means convincing, medical science and research have proved that a healthy lifestyle makes a difference to the health of our brain. Some of the critical factors that may reduce the impact of dementia are quite outstanding to most people at this point, yet it merits emphasizing them. Avoid

Smoking. Not smoking prevents the beginning of dementia. It additionally brings down the danger of a few other smoker related diseases. Inactive smoking can, in any case, be a problem, however, has been incredibly reduced by the introduction of smoking bans in the workplace and open zones.

When you quit smoking the body begins fixing itself straightaway regardless of to what extent you have been a smoker. At the point when the body is all around maintained and cared for, it will run effectively well into old age.

Alcohol Consumption. Nobody can dictate precisely how much alcohol someone else should drink, yet the standard drinks principle does set guidelines for dependable drinking. Alcohol like smoking has a whole raft of associated diseases that are very much documented.

Physical Exercise. Stoutness is presently looming as the following health-related fiasco; this is stunning when you believe that it is a preventable disease. Strolling, cycling or cardiovascular exercise reinforces the heart and the blood vessels to the brain. Apart from keeping you physically fit, it encourages the brain to become more keen and more alarm.

Adequate Sleep. A solid night's sleep is essential for good health. This is the first time the body can recuperate and revive itself. While it is conceivable to make do with minimal rest in the short term, it isn't savvy to do it all the time.

After some time, sleep deprivation can cause significant health problems. And researchers are currently studying the impact that lack of sleep can have on the brain. They have proved that in the short term, it can influence judgment, mood, and the capacity to learn and hold information.

Lack of sleep can likewise disrupt the immune system, and long term it can lead to diseases, for example, heart disease, hypertension, and diabetes.

Healthy Eating Habits. A healthy diet should include new wholesome food and practically no processed food. Keep your fluid levels topped up with water as opposed to soda pops or sweet squeezes.

The entire diet issue can be a bit of a minefield. It merely is preposterous to expect to recommend an eating plan that suits everybody. Do your research, don't get taken in by extravagant marketing and remember that supplements are only that; they are to supplement a diet that is deficient of a particular vitamin or mineral. They can't compensate for the lack of a balanced diet. Attempt not eating on the run, bite food altogether and if conceivable eat at a table in a comfortable position. It is never past the point where it is possible to make changes to your lifestyle.

Lifestyle Changes.

The good thing about exercising the brain is the sheer number of exercises or activities that are accessible. Anyway, it is essential to different exercises, so they don't become repetition. Of course, brain exercises don't need to be exercised in the strictest terms, any activity that involves believing is an exercise in itself. An activity which involves learning something new is good for the brain, even a simple task being done out of the blue engages the mind into deduction mode. Problem explaining is a form of brain exercise, particularly complex problems with multiple arrangements. It could be argued that people who work or lead a bustling life don't need to do brain exercises, yet it depends on the amount they extend the brain. Tasks which at the outset may have seemed complex become more comfortable, so the brain doesn't work so hard. Anyone who has ever learned to drive can relate to this. At first, it is alarming attempting to remember every one of the moves, mainly if it is a manual drive. Anyway, it before long becomes so characteristic that you hardly need to consider it, it is a bit like being on automatic pilot. It is almost as though the brain is stating, "Wake me when something occurs." The old saying "Use it or lose it" has a lot of merits where the brain is concerned, so exercising it makes sense. Albeit many people consider brain exercises in terms of Sudoku, Scrabble, or chess, it is a much broader subject out and out. For anyone considering doing these types of activities and wondering what would be best here is a short outline that may help. Above all else, the exercises can be grouped into three main classifications.

1) Games. Brain exercises that are only that brain exercises, and that's it.

Games, for example, Scrabble, Sudoku, chess and similar, are ideal because apart from exercising the brain, they are a form of enjoyment or unwinding. They are compact and should be possible anyplace whenever, ideal in the circumstances like travel when one needs to stick around. Mobile platforms presently make it easier than at any other time. I could never get anyone to play scrabble with me, yet nowadays I play against the computer at whatever point I need.

Of course, if any of these games are notched up to competition level that involves a more fabulous workout for the brain.

2) Brain exercises as a result.

This happens when you take up another premium that has a learning bend. If for example, you became interested in astronomy and wanted to learn about it, your brain would need to process all the new information. This is an incredible method to exercise the brain regularly.

As our life becomes more dominated by innovation, it is significant to secure aptitudes which enable us to exploit the electronic age. Since computer innovation is sophisticated, it involves a considerable learning bend. Chris has dependably been into computers. However, I put off utilizing one for a considerable length of time since everything seemed excessively hard. Luckily it is never past the point of no return, and now I have one of my own and don't comprehend what I would do without it!

3) Brain exercises with a reason.

This happens when you undertake a task because of an end goal. You might do a college course to get a degree or learn a language to go voyaging. Maybe you need a complete change of profession and need to learn another arrangement of aptitudes. These types of activities appeal to people who like a test or who are hoping to make changes in their life. Expanding numbers of older people or retirees are moving in this direction since they believe they need more out of life than to lounge around doing perplexes on a permanent premise. In his book "The brain that changes itself,"

Norman Doidge M.D. Refers to the instance of Dr. Stanley Karansky who practiced as an anesthesiologist until he retired at age 70. Retirement didn't suit him, so he restrained himself as a family doctor and worked until he was 80. Not all that many years back the "Masters Games" were introduced because so many older people were participating in a competitive game. Watching contestants aged in the nineties competing in marathons and swimming races would have seemed impossible to our parents and grandparents. We currently acknowledge it as usual and as we learn more about what the brain is fit for who comprehends what the future will bring. Brain health isn't only a fad it is digging in for the long haul, and nobody will scrutinize the fact that our brain, similar to the remainder of our body needs regular exercise and a proper diet.

Brahmanism dates back to containing sacred scriptures called "the Vedas". These scriptures contained instructions and incantations. It was in the oldest text "Rg-Veda" from the scriptures that the word Yoga first appeared, this was nearly 5000 years ago. The fourth text called "Atharva-Veda" contains mainly spells for magical rites and health cures many of which use medicinal plants. This text provided the average person with the spells and incantations to use in their everyday life and this practice of "Veda" can still be seen in the streets of India today. The Bhagavad-Gita, another ancient work on spiritual life describes itself as a yoga treatise, although it uses the word Yoga as a spiritual means. It was from this literature that Patanjali's "eight limbs of yoga" were developed. Yoga Sutra's are primarily concerned with developing the "nature of the mind" and I will explain more of this in the next section.The Breadth ....

The vratyas, a group of fertility priests who worshipped Rudra, god of the wind would attempt to imitate the sound of the wind through their singing. They found that they could produce the sound through the control of their breath and through this practice of breath control was formed "Pranayama". Pranayama is the practice of breath control in yoga.
The Paths ....The Upanishads, which are the sacred revelations of ancient Hinduism developed the two disciplines of karma yoga,

the path of action and jnana yoga, the path of knowledge. The paths were developed to help the student liberate from suffering and eventually gain enlightenment. The teaching from the Upanishads differed from that of the Vedas. The Vedas demanded external offerings to the gods in order to have an abundant, happy life. The Upanishads through the practice of Karma yoga focused on the internal sacrifice of the ego in order to liberate from suffering. Instead of the sacrifice of crops and animals (external) it was the sacrifice of the inner ego that would become the basic philosophy, thus yoga became known as the path of renunciation. Yoga shares some characteristics also with Buddhism that can be traced back through history. During the sixth century B.C., Buddhism also stresses the importance of Meditation and the practice of physical postures. Siddharta Gautama was the first Buddhist to actually study Yoga. What is Yoga Sutra and how did the Philosophy of Yoga develop ?Yoga Sutra is a compilation of 195 statements which essentially provide an ethical guide for living moral life and incorporating the science of yoga into it. An Indian sage called Patanjali was believed to have collated this over 2000 years ago and it has become the cornerstone for classical yoga philosophy.The word sutra means literally "a thread" and is used to denote a particular form of written and oral communication. Because of the brus☐ue style the sutras are written in the student must rely on a guru to interpret the philosophy contained within each one. The meaning within each of the sutras can be tailored to the student's particular needs.The Yoga Sutra is a system of yoga however there is not a single description of a posture or asana in it! Patanjali developed a guide for living the right life. The core of his teachings is the "eightfold path of yoga" or "the eight limbs of Patanjali" . These are Patanjali's suggestions for living a better life through yoga. Posture and breath control, the two fundamental practices of yoga are described as the third and fourth limbs in Patanjali's eight-limbed path to self-realisation. The third practice of the postures make up today's modern yoga. When you join a yoga class you may find that   is   all   you   need   to   suit   your   lifestyle.

The eight limbs of yoga

1. The yamas (restraints),

These are like "Morals" you live your life by: Your social conduct:

o Nonviolence (ahimsa) - To not hurt a living creature

O Truth and honesty (satya) - To not lie o Nonstealing (asteyal)

O Nonlust (brahmacharya) - avoid meaningless sexual encounters - moderation in sex and all things.

O Nonpossessiveness or non-greed (aparigraha) - don't hoard, free yourself from greed and material desires

2.   niyamas (observances),

These are how we treat ourselves, our inner discipline:

O purity (shauca). Achieving purity through the practice of the five Yamas. Treating your body as a temple and looking after it.

O Contentment (santosha). Find happiness in what you have and what you do. Take responsibility for where you are, seek happiness in the moment and choose to grow.

O Austerity (tapas): Develop self discipline. Show discipline in body, speech, and mind to aim for a higher spiritual purpose.

O Study of the sacred text (svadhyaya). Education. Study books relevant to you which inspire and teach you.

O Living with an awareness of the Divine (ishvara-pranidhana). Be devoted to whatever is your god or whatever you see as the divine.

3.   asana (postures) -

These are the postures of yoga:

O To create a supple body in order to sit for a lengthy time and still the mind. If you can control the body you can also control the mind. Patanjali and other ancient yogis used asana to prepare the body for meditation. Just the practice of the yoga postures can benefit one's health. It can be started at any time and any age. As we grow older we stiffen, do you remember the last time you may have squatted down to pick something up and how you felt? Imagine as you age into your fifties, sixties, seventies and on being able to still touch your toes or balance on one leg. Did you know that the majority of injuries sustained by the elderly are from falls? We tend to lose our balance as we grow older and to practice something that will help this is surely a benefit.

The fourth limb, breath control is a good vehicle to use if you are interested in learning meditation and relaxation ...

4. pranayama (breathing) - the control of breath:

inhalation, retention of breath, and exhalation

O The practice of breathing makes it easier to concentrate and meditate. Prana is the energy that exists everywhere, it is the life force that flows through each of us through our breath.

5. pratyahara (withdrawal of senses),

O Pratyahara is a withdrawal of the senses. It occurs during meditation, breathing exercises, or the practice of yoga postures. When you master Pratyahara you will be able to focus and concentrate and not be distracted by outward sensory.

6. dharana (concentration), - teaching the mind to focus.

O When concentrating there is no sense of time. The aim is to still the mind e.g. fixing the mind on one object and pushing any thoughts. True dharana is when the mind can concentrate effortlessly.

7. Dhyani (meditation), - the state of meditation

O Concentration (dharana) leads to the state of meditation. In meditation, one has a heightened sense of awareness and is one with the universe. It is being unaware of any distractions.

8. samadhi (absorption), - absolute bliss

O Absolute bliss is the ultimate goal of meditation. This is a state of union with yourself and your god or the devine, this is when you and the universe are one. All eight limbs work together: The first five are about the body and brain- yama, niyama asana, pranayama, and pratyahara - these are the foundations of yoga and provide a platform for a spiritual life. The last three are about reconditioning the mind. They were developed to help the practitioner to attain enlightenment or oneness with Spirit.

How do you choose the type of yoga right for you?
The type of yoga you choose to practice is entirely an individual preference and thus why we are looking into here to help you start. Some types hold the postures longer, some move through them quicker. Some styles focus on body alignment, others differ in the rhythm and selection of postures, meditation and spiritual realization. All are adaptable to the student's physical situation. You therefore need to determine what Yoga style by your individual psychological and physical needs. You may just want a vigorous workout, want to focus on developing your flexibility or balance. Do you want more focus on meditation or just the health aspects? Some schools teach relaxation, some focus on strength and agility, and others are more aerobic. suggest you try a few different classes in your area. I have noticed that even between teachers within a certain style, there can be differences in how the student enjoys the class. It is important to find a teacher that you feel comfortable with to truly enjoy and therefore create longevity in what you practice. Once you start learning the postures and adapting them for your body you may feel comfortable to do practice at home as well! All yoga types have sequences that can be practiced to work different parts of your body. To A fifteen minute practice in the morning may be your start to the day. Your body will feel strong and lithe within no time and with knowledge, the choice is there for you to develop your own routines. The two major systems of yoga are Hatha and Yoga Raja Yoga. Raja yoga is based on the "Eight Limbs of Yoga" developed by Pananjali in the Yoga Sutras. Raja is part of the classical Indian System of Hindu Philosophy. Hatha yoga, also Hatha vidya is a particular system of Yoga founded by Swatmarama, a yogic sage of the 15th centry in India. Swatmarama compiled the "Hatha Yoga Pradipika", which introduced the system of Hatha Yoga. Hatha yoga is derived from a number of different traditions. It comes from the traditions of

Buddhism which include the Hinayana (narrow path) and Mahayana (great path). It also comes from the traditions of Tantra which include Sahajayana (spontaneous path) and Vajrayana (concerning matters of sexuality). Within Hatha yoga there are various branches or styles of yoga. This form of yoga works through the physical medium of the body using postures, breathing exercises and cleansing practices. The Hatha Yoga of Swatmarama differs from the Raja Yoga of Patanjali in that it focuses on Shatkarma, "the purification of the physical" as a path leading to "purification of the mind" and "vital energy". Patanjali begins with "purification of the mind and spirit" and then "the body" through postures and breath.There are approximately forty-four major schools of Yoga and many others which also lay claim to being Yogic. Some of the major schools are Raja Yoga and Hatha Yoga (as mentioned above). There are also Pranayama Yoga and Kundalini Yoga which stem from Hatha. Jnana, Karma, Bhakti, Astanga and Iyengar stem from Raja.

The Yoga Styles that stem from Hatha include:

Pranayama Yoga
The word pranayama means prana, energy and ayama, stretch. Breath regulation, prolongation, expansion, length, stretch and control describes the action of pranayama yoga. Some Pranayama breath controls are included in the Hatha Yoga practices of a general nature (to correct breathing difficulties). This school of yoga is entirely built around the concept of Prana (life's energy). There are about different postures of which a lot of these are based around or similar to physical breathing exercises. Pranayama also denotes cosmic power, or the power of the entire universe which manifests itself as conscious living being in us through the phenomenon of breathing.

Kundalini Yoga
Kundalini yoga is in the tradition of Yogi Bhajan who brought the style to the west in 1969. It is a highly spiritual approach to hatha yoga involving chanting, meditation, breathing techniques all used to raise the kundalini energy which is located at the base of the spine.

The Yoga Styles that stem from Raja include:
Raja Yoga/Ashtanga Yoga
Raja means royal or kingly. It is based on directing one's life force to bring the mind and emotions into balance. By doing so the attention can then be focused on the object of the meditation, namely the Devine. Raja Yoga or Ashtanga Yoga is one of the four major Yogic paths of Hinduism. The others are Karma Yoga, Jnana Yoga and Bhakti Yoga. Raja or Ashtanga are derived from the "eight limbs of Yoga" philosophy composed by Patanjali.

Power Yoga
Power Yoga has been devised through the teachings of Sri K. Pattabhi Jois, a renowned Sanskrit scholar who inspired Western Yogis with his Ashtanga Yoga Style and philosophies. It is therefore often referred to as the western version of India's Ashtanga yoga. Power yoga is vigorous and athletic and is therefore very popular with men. It works with the student's mental attitude and perspective and incorporates the eight limbs of yoga into practice.

Jnana Yoga

Jnana (sometimes spelled "Gnana") means wisdom and a Jnani is a wise man. Sometimes referred to as the" yogi of discernment". This form of yoga focuses on studying inner life and adhyatmic subjects, the practice of certain relaxations and contemplative, meditative kriyas. The main purpose of jnana meditation is to withdraw the mind and emotions from perceiving life and oneself in a deluded way so that one may behold and live in attunement with reality or spirit. This form of yoga focuses on meditation to work towards transformation and enlightenment.

Karma Yoga
Karma means "action". Karma yoga is based around the discipline of action based on the teachings of Bhagavad Gita, a holy scripture of Hinduism. This yoga of selfless service focuses on the adherence to duty (dharma) while remaining detached from the reward. Karma is the sum total of our acts, both in the present life and in the preceding births.

Bhakti Yoga
Bhaki yoga has many phases to it's practice. Bhaki means "devotion" and Guna Bhaki is to worship according to your nature. A practitioner of Bhakta Yoga is not limited to any one culture or religious denomination, the approach is more to the inner life rather than the wholly devotional. The self within worships the self of the universal nature. Bhaki yoga is the state of being in contact with our existence and being and the existence and being of all things. It doesn't matter if you believe in something or you don't the only Duality is the openness to the

mind and heart, unexpected and unknown. Those who have read about Quantum physics where each and every atom in the universe is connected to the underlying reality will be able to liken this to the philosophy behind Bhaki yoga.

Iyengar Yoga
Iyengar Yoga was developed in India by B.K.S Iyengar, born 14th December, 1918. At the age of 16, he was introduced to yoga by his Guru Sri T. Krishnamacharya. Iyengar Yoga is now one of the most popular styles practiced in the west. Instructors are very knowledgeable about the anatomy and precise body place for each posture. There is less focus on pranayama or breathing techniques and mediation and thus why the practice is popular in the west. Iyengar Yoga emphasizes more on the correct placement of the feet to ensure the spine and the hips are in alignment. Iyengar has developed many different props and techniques to cater for individuals in their practice.

Other Styles

Integral Yoga or Purna Yoga
Integral yoga is a yoga of synthesis, harmonizing the paths of karma, jnana and bhakti yogas. It was developed by Swami Satchidananda. It is also considered a synthesis between Vedanta (Indian system of philosophy) and Tantra (Asian beliefs and practices using the principle that the divine energy creates and maintains the universe, channelling the energy within the human microcosm). It also been explained as a synthesis between Eastern and Western approaches to spirituality. Postures are

gentler than other forms of yoga and classes normally end with extended periods of deep relaxation, breathing and meditation. Integral Yoga is an all round approach to hatha yoga.

Sivananda Yoga
Sivananda yoga offers a gentle approach. It includes meditation, chanting and deep relaxation in each session. Students are encouraged to be healthy which includes being vegetarian. Bikrams YogaBikrams yoga was founded by Bikram Choudhury who was taught by Bishni Ghosh the brother of Paramahansa Yogananda. Bikrams Yoga is taught generally in a room the temperature set between 95 and 105 degrees. The heat helps soften the muscles and ligaments. There are approximately 26 postures and this yoga produces a real workout because of the heat is quite intense. This yoga therefore places more emphasis on the physical performance of the postures, not the sides of relaxation and meditation.

Some of the Great Teachers...
All styles share a common lineage. The founders of two of the major styles of yoga Raja/Ashtanga and Avenger were all students of the same great teacher named Krishnamacharya. Shri T. Krishnamacharya,was born in the village of Muchukunte, Karnataka State, in 1888. His formal Education, largely in Sanskrit, included Degrees from several universities in North India. He studied for seven years under a distinguished yogi in western Tibet: Rama Mohana Brahmachari who instructed him the

therapeutic use of asanas & pranayama. Then he returned to South India and established a school of yoga in the palace of the Maharajah of Mysore. He passed away at the age of 101 years in 1988. Integral Yoga and Sivananda Yoga were also founded by students of another great teacher named Sivananda. Swami Sivananda Saraswati was born Kuppuswamy in Pattamadai, Tamil Nadu, India. A Hindu by birth, he is a well-known proponent of yoga and vedanta (a principal branch of Hindu philosophy). He is reputed to have written over 300 books, on these and related subjects, during his life. In 1936 he founded the new religious movement "The Divine Life Society" on the bank of the holy Ganges River. He died on the 14th July, 1963.

So which type is right for you?

These are not all the types of yoga available, however you can see from the short explanations of each that Yoga practice can differ dramatically. Each one makes use of the physical postures and breathing to strengthen the body for meditation, an inherent part of yoga practice. This is where it is important for the student to understand what they want out of their yoga practice and choose a style which will cater for this. If you try one and don't think it is physical enough, try another as it will be totally different. If you start one that is too demanding than again switch around until you find the practice for you. Some of us want to just work on body and some want more focus on a method of searching for self realisation, whatever the reason I am sure there are enough styles out their and more developing each day to cater for our needs. You are never too old to start yoga, I have met people in their seventies starting for the first time and experiencing life changing affects. If you've ever sat and watched your cat or dog awake in the morning what is the first thing they do? stretch. If we stop for just a moment and watch what we can learn from nature and the animal kingdom we will realize that just the simple act of stretching has been lost somewhere through our evolution. The table below shows the rating between 1 and 10 I have given to explain the degree of Physical and degree of Meditation/Relaxation in each Yoga practice (10 being the highest)

Name of Yoga Physical Rating Meditation & Relaxation Rating

Pranayama Yoga 4 8

Kundalini Yoga 6 8

Raja Yoga/Ashtanga Yoga 10 6

Power Yoga 10 2

Jnana Yoga 6 8

Karma Yoga 6 8

Bhakti Yoga 6 8

Iyengar Yoga 8 4

Integral Yoga or Purna Yoga 6 8

Sivananda Yoga 6 8

Bikrams Yoga 10 (due to the heat) 2

Can We Have Both?

It's easy to understand why John Friend highly recommends the book Yoga Body: The Origins of Modern Posture Yoga "for all sincere students of yoga." Because, Mark Singleton's thesis is a well researched expose of how modern hatha yoga, or "posture practice," as he terms it, has changed within and after the practice left India. But the book is mainly about how yoga transformed in India itself in the last 150 years. How yoga's main, modern proponents-T. Krishnamacharya and his students, K. Patttabhi Jois and B. K. S. Iyengar-mixed their homegrown hatha yoga practices with European gymnastics. This was how many Indian yogis coped with modernity: Rather than remaining in the caves of the Himalayas, they moved to the city and embraced the oncoming European cultural trends. They especially embraced its more "esoteric forms of gymnastics," including the influential Swedish techniques of Ling (1766-1839). Singleton uses the word yoga as a homonym to explain the main goal of his thesis. That is, he emphasizes that the word yoga has multiple meanings, depending on who uses the term. This emphasis is in itself a worthy enterprise for students of everything yoga; to comprehend and accept that your yoga may not be the same kind of yoga as my yoga. Simply, that there are many paths of yoga. In that regard, John Friend is absolutely right: this is by far the most comprehensive study of the culture and history of the influential yoga lineage that runs from T. Krishnamacharya's humid and hot palace studio in Mysore to Bikram's artificially heated studio in Hollywood. Singleton's study on "postural yoga" makes up the bulk of the book. But he also devotes some pages to outline the history of "traditional" yoga, from Patanjali to the Shaiva Tantrics who, based on much earlier yoga traditions, compiled the hatha yoga tradition in the middle ages and penned the famous yoga text books the Hatha Yoga Pradipika and the Geranda Samhita. It is while doing these examinations that Singleton gets into water much hotter than a Bikram sweat. Thus I hesitate in giving Singleton a straight A for his otherwise excellent dissertation. Singleton claims his project is solely the study of modern posture yoga. If he had stuck to that project alone, his book would have been great and received only accolades. But unfortunately, he commits the same blunder so many modern hatha yogis do. All yoga styles are fine, these hatha yogis say. All homonyms are equally good and valid, they claim. Except that homonym, which the cultural relativist hatha yogis perceive as an arrogant version of yoga. Why? Because its adherents, the traditionalists, claim it is a deeper, more spiritual and traditional from of yoga. This kind of ranking, thinks Singleton, is counterproductive and a waste of time. Georg Feuerstein disagrees. Undoubtedly the most prolific and well-respected yoga scholar outside India today, he is one of those traditionalists who holds yoga to be an integral practice-a body, mind, spirit practice. So how does Feuerstein's integral yoga homonym differ from the non-integral modern posture yoga homonym presented to us by Singleton? Simply put, Feuerstein's remarkable writings on yoga have focused on the holistic practice of yoga. On the whole shebang of practices that traditional yoga developed over the past 5000 plus years: asanas, pranayama (breathing exercises), chakra (subtle energy centers), kundalini (spiritual energy), bandhas (advanced body locks), mantras, mudras (hand gestures), etc. Hence, while posture yoga primarily focuses on the physical body, on doing postures, integral yoga includes both the physical and the subtle body and involves a whole plethora of physical, mental and spiritual practices hardly ever practiced in any of today's modern yoga studios. would not have bothered to bring all this up had it not been for the fact that Singleton mentioned Feuerstein in a critical light in his book's "Concluding Reflections." In other words, it is strategically important for Singleton to critique Feuerstein's interpretation of yoga, a form of yoga which happens to pretty much coincide with my own. Singleton writes: "For some, such as best-selling yoga scholar Georg Feuerstein, the modern fascination with postural yoga can only be a perversion of the authentic yoga of tradition." Then Singleton quotes Feuerstein, who writes that when yoga reached Western shores it "was gradually stripped of its spiritual orientation and remodeled into fitness training." Singleton then correctly points out that yoga had already started this fitness change in India. He also correctly points out that fitness yoga is not apposed to any "spiritual" enterprise of yoga. But that is not exactly Feuerstein's point: he simply points out how the physical exercise part of modern yoga lacks a deep "spiritual orientation." And that is a crucial difference. Then Singleton exclaims that Feuerstein's assertions misses the "deeply spiritual orientation of some modern bodybuilding and women's fitness training in the harmonial gymnastics tradition." While I think I am quite clear about what Feuerstein means by "deeply spiritual," I am still not sure what Singleton means by it from just reading Yoga Body. And that makes an intelligent comparison difficult. Hence why did Singleton bring this up in his concluding arguments in a book devoted to physical postures? Surely to make a point.

Since he did make a point about it, I would like to respond. According to Feuerstein, the goal of yoga is enlightenment (Samadhi), not physical fitness, not even spiritual physical fitness. Not a better, slimmer physique, but a better chance at spiritual liberation. For him, yoga is primarily a spiritual practice involving deep postures, deep study and deep meditation. Even though postures are an integral part of traditional yoga, enlightenment is possible even without the practice of posture yoga, indisputably proven by such sages as Ananda Mai Ma, Ramana Maharishi, Nisargadatta Maharaj, and others. The broader question about the goal of yoga, from the point of view of traditional yoga is this: is it possible to attain enlightenment through the practice of fitness yoga alone? The answer: Not very easy. Not even likely. Not even by practicing the kind of fitness yoga Singleton claims is "spiritual." According to integral yoga, the body is the first and outer layer of the mind. Enlightenment, however, takes place in and beyond the fifth and innermost layer of the subtle body, or kosa, not in the physical body. Hence, from this particular perspective of yoga, fitness yoga has certain limits, simply because it cannot alone deliver the desired results. Similarily, Feuerstein and all us other traditionalists (oh, those darn labels!) are simply saying that if your goal is enlightenment, then fitness yoga probably won't do the trick. You can stand on your head and do power yoga from dawn to midnight, but you still won't be enlightened. Hence, they designed sitting yoga postures (padmasana, siddhasana, viirasana, etc) for such particular purposes. Indeed, they spent more time sitting still in meditation over moving about doing postures, as it was the sitting practices which induced the desired trance states of enlightenment, or Samadhi. In other words, you can be enlightened without ever practicing the varied hatha postures, but you probably won't get enlightened by just practicing these postures alone, no matter how "spiritual" those postures are. These are the kinds of layered insights and perspectives I sorely missed while reading Yoga Body. Hence his criticism of Feuerstein seems rather shallow and kneejerk. Singleton's sole focus on describing the physical practice and history of modern yoga is comprehensive, probably quite accurate, and rather impressive, but his insistence that there are "deeply spiritual" aspects of modern gymnastics and posture yoga misses an important point about yoga. Namely, that our bodies are only as spiritual as we are, from that space in our hearts, deep within and beyond the body. Yoga Body thus misses a crucial point many of us have the right to claim, and without having to be criticized for being arrogant or mean-minded: that yoga is primarily a holistic practice, in which the physical body is seen as the first layer of a series of ascending and all-embracing layers of being-from body to mind to spirit. And that ultimately, even the body is the dwelling place of Spirit. In sum, the body is the sacred temple of Spirit. And where does this yoga perspective hail from? According to Feuerstein, "It underlies the entire Tantric tradition, notably the schools of hatha yoga, which are an offshoot of

Tantrism." In Tantra it is clearly understood that the human being is a three-tiered being-physical, mental and spiritual. Hence, the Tantrics very skillfully and carefully developed practices for all three levels of being. From this ancient perspective, it is very gratifying to see how the more spiritual, all-embracing tantric and yogic practices such as hatha yoga, mantra meditation, breathing exercises, ayurveda, kirtan, and scriptural study are increasingly becoming integral features of many modern yoga studios. So, to answer the question in the title of this article. Can we have both a limber physique and a sacred spirit while practicing yoga? Yes, of course we can. Yoga is not either/or. Yoga is yes/and. The more holistic our yoga practice becomes-that is, the more spiritual practice is added to our posture practice-the more these two seemingly opposite poles-the body and the spirit-will blend and unify. Unity was, after all, the goal of ancient Tantra. Perhaps soon someone will write a book about this new, ever-growing homonym of global yoga? Mark Singleton's Yoga Body is not such a book. But a book about this, shall we call it, neo-traditional, or holistic form of yoga would certainly be an interesting cultural exploration.

Origin and Background

Yoga is an age-old science made up of different disciplines of mind and body. It has originated in India 2500 years ago and is still effective in bringing overall health and well being to any person who does it regularly. The word yoga is based upon a

Sanskrit verb Yuja. It means to connect, to culminate or to concur. It's the culmination of mind and body or the culmination of Jiva and Shiva (soul and the universal spirit). It's also a culmination of Purush and Prakriti (Yin and Yang). The term Yoga has a very broad scope. There are several schools or systems of Yoga. Dnyanayoga (Yoga through knowledge), Bhaktiyoga (Yoga through devotion), Karmayoga (Yoga through action), Rajayoga (Royal or supreme Yoga) and Hathayoga (Yoga by balancing opposite principles of body). All of these schools of Yoga are not necessarily very different from each other. They are rather like threads of the same cloth, entangled into each other. For thousands of years, Yoga has been looked upon as an effective way of self-improvement and spiritual enlightenment. All these systems essentially have this same purpose; only the ways of achieving it are little different for each of them. In its most popular form, the term Yoga has come to associate with the last of these systems which is Hathayoga. For the purpose of this article too, the term Yoga is used with the same meaning. Although, when it comes to Philosophy of Yoga, which is at the end of this article, the term Yoga will have a broader scope.

Asana and Pranayama
Let's take a detailed look at the main two components of Hathayoga i.e. Asana and Pranayama.

a) Asana:
Asana means acquiring a body posture and maintaining it as long as one's body allows. Asana, when done rightly according to the

rules discussed above, render enormous physical and psychological benefits. Asana are looked upon as the preliminary step to Pranayama. With the practice of Asana there is a balancing of opposite principles in the body and psyche. It also helps to get rid of inertia. Benefits of Asana are enhanced with longer maintenance of it. Asana should be stable, steady and pleasant. Here is the summary of general rules to be followed for doing Asana.

Summary of rules:

1.   Normal breathing

2.   Focused stretching

3.   Stable and pleasant postures (sthiram sukham asanam)

4.   Minimal efforts (Prayatnay shaithilyam)

5.   No comparisons or competition with others

6.   No jerks or rapid actions. Maintain a slow and steady tempo.

Each asana has its own benefits and a few common benefits such as stability, flexibility, better hormonal secretion, feeling refreshed and rejuvenated. It's a misconception that an Asana (Yoga stretch) has to be difficult to do in order to be beneficial. Many of the easiest Asana render most of the common benefits of Yoga to their fullest. Besides, the beauty of Yoga is in the fact that at a not-so-perfect level most of the benefits are still available. That means even a beginner benefits from Yoga as much as an expert. In their quest to find a solution to the miseries of human body and mind, the founders of Yoga found part of their answers in the nature. They watched the birds and animals stretching their bodies in particular fashion to get rid of the inertia and malaise. Based upon these observations, they created Yoga stretches and named them after the birds or animals or fish that inspired these stretches. For example, matsyasana (fish pose), makarasana (crocodile pose), shalabhasana (grasshopper pose), bhujangasana (cobra pose), marjarasana (cat pose), mayurasana (peacock pose), vrischikasana (scorpion pose), gomukhasana (cow's mouth pose), parvatasana (mountain pose), vrikshasana (tree pose) etc. Many of the Asana can be broadly categorized based upon the type of pressure on the abdomen. Most of the forward bending Asana are positive pressure Asana as they put positive pressure on the stomach by crunching it e.g. Pashchimatanasana, Yogamudra (Yoga symbol pose), Hastapadasana (hand and feet pose), Pavanmuktasana (wind free pose) etc. The backward bending Asana are the negative pressure Asana as they take pressure away from the abdomen e.g. Dhanurasana (bow pose), Bhujangasana (cobra pose), Naukasana (boat pose) etc. Both types of Asana give excellent stretch to the back and abdomen and strengthen both these organs. Alternating between positive and negative pressure on the same area of the body intensifies and enhances blood circulation in that area. The muscle group in use gets more supply of oxygen and blood due to the pressure on that spot. E.g. in Yogamudra (symbol of Yoga), the lower abdomen gets positive pressure due to which Kundalini is awakened. Hastapadasana refreshes all nerves in the back of the legs and also in the back. As a result you feel fresh and rejuvenated. Vakrasana gives a good massage to the pancreas and liver and hence is recommended for diabetic patients.

2.   Pranayama

Practicing Pranayama is one of the ways of getting rid of mental disturbances and physical ill health. Pranayama means controlled and prolonged span of breath. Prana means breath. It also means life force. Ayama means controlling or elongation. Just like a pendulum requires twice long to come back to its original position, the exhalations in Pranayama are twice longer than the inhalations. The main purpose of Pranayama is to bring mental stability and restrain desires by controlling breathing. Breathing is a function of autonomous nervous system. By bringing the involuntary process of breathing under control of mind, the scope of volition is broadened. Pranayama is a bridge between Bahiranga (exoteric) Yoga and Antaranga (introspective or esoteric) Yoga. A body that has become stable by Asana and has been cleansed by Kriya (cleansing processes) is ready for Pranayama. On the other hand Pranayama prepares the mind and body for meditational and spiritual practice of Yoga such as Dhyana, Dharana and Samadhi. On physical level, practice of Pranayama increases blood in oxygen, subsequently refreshing and rejuvenating the brain and the nerves. Here are a few physical benefits of Pranayama. a. Lungs, chest, diaphragm become stronger and healthier.

b. Capacity of lungs is increased.

c. Slow changing pressure creates a form of massage to all organs in the stomach cavity.

d.   Purifies blood by increasing blood's capacity to absorb more oxygen.

e.   Brain functions better with more oxygen in the blood.

f.   Neuromuscular coordination improves.

g.   Body becomes lean and the skin glows.
There are 8 main Pranayama namely, Ujjayi, Suryabhedan, Sitkari, Shitali, Bhastrika, Bhramari, Murchha, Plavini. Among these, Ujjayi is the most popular Pranayama. Pranayama consists of 4 parts in the following order:

1)   Puraka (Controlled inhalation)

2)   Abhyantara Kumbhaka (Holding breath in)
3)   Rechaka (Controlled exhalation)
4) Bahya Kumbhaka (Holding breath out).

The ratio of these parts to each other is generally 1:4:2:4 with a few exceptions. Patanjali's Yogasutra agrees with this ratio along with many other scriptures. For the purpose of overall well-being, practicing the first three parts is sufficient. A spiritual practitioner generally practices all four parts including the last one i.e. Bahya Kumbhaka. Such a practitioner also does many more repetitions than someone who does it for general health and well-being. Out of the four parts of Pranayama, it's the Abhyantara Kumbhaka that is essentially identified with Pranayama. There is one more Kumbhaka that happens spontaneously and is called Keval Kumbhaka. Bandha (Locks) are very crucial to the practice of

Pranayama. Mulabandha (locking the anus), Jalandharbandha (locking the throat area or jugular notch), Udiyanabandha (locking the abdomen or diaphragm) and Jivhabandha (locking the tongue) are the four locks that are performed during Pranayama. Depending upon the purpose of Pranayama (spiritual or general health), locks are performed. Mulabandha, Jalandharbandha and Udiyanabandha are the common Bandha performed by everyone. Jivhabandha is mandatory only if done for spiritual purposes.

Characteristics of Yoga

Let's take a look at some of the chief characteristics of Yoga.

1)   Yoga is not an exercise.

To understand the concept of Yoga one must keep in mind that the positions in Yoga are not exercises but bodily stretches and maintenance of stretches. You may describe Yoga in terms of Yogic stretches or Yogic practices. Acquiring a body position by stretching the muscles and then maintaining this position as long as one's body allows, that is what Yogic stretches are. Yoga requires very smooth and controlled motions and a slow steady tempo. To achieve this one needs to have total concentration of mind while doing Yoga. The movements in Yoga are smooth, slow and controlled. Comparison with others is greatly discouraged. Doing something beyond one's capacity just out of competition generally results in hurting one's body and hence is greatly discouraged. Breathing in Yoga remains steady unlike many aerobic exercises. Yoga is also Isotonic unlike bodybuilding exercises, which are isometric in nature. In isotonic stretches, length of the muscles increases while tone stays the same as opposed to the isometric exercises in which length of the muscles stays the same while the tone changes. In Isotonic stretches, body is stretched in a particular manner and maintained that way for some time.

2) Longer maintenance and fewer repetitions (as per the body's capacity).

Benefits of Yoga are enhanced with the maintenance of a body stretch. Longer the maintenance better will be the effect. However one cannot force oneself into maintaining the stretch longer than the body can bear. Each and every position is pleasant and stable (Sthiram Sukham Asanam). Sthiram means steady. Sukham means pleasant and Asanam means a body posture or position. The right position for you is that in which your body remains steady (sthiram) and which is pleasant and comfortable to you (sukham). The moment a stretch becomes unbearable and uncomfortable and the body starts shaking, one needs to come out of that position in a very slow, smooth and controlled manner. There will be more repetitions and shorter maintenance for a beginner. With more practice, the repetitions will be fewer and maintenance will be longer. After doing Yoga one should only feel pleasant and fresh and nothing else. If you feel tired or fatigued or any part of your body aches, it only means that you have tried beyond your capacity.

3) Trust your body. Apply minimum efforts:

With the practice of Yoga, you also learn to trust your body's capacity to progress in terms of flexibility without conscious efforts. As long as the aim is in mind and the body is stretched only to its current capacity, the flexibility develops on its own. One needs to just focus on breath, focus on the present state of the body pose and enjoy that pose as long as it feels comfortable. 'Prayatnay Shaithilyam' means minimum efforts. Although there is an ideal position described and desired for each asana, no one is forced into attaining the ideal position. Yoga is done with the trust that flexibility is acquired after a continuous and regular practice. There is a message here and that is to have faith in the unknown. This message along with the improved endocrine function, better muscle tone, calmer mind and increased positive outlook can be enormously beneficial for recovery from any illness.

4) Focused stretching:

The ability to stretch or pressure one muscle group while relaxing the rest of the body is called focused stretching. For example if a particular Asana is based upon stretching the stomach as the main muscle group (the pivotal muscles), then the rest of the body is relaxed while the stomach is stretched or pressured. One has to watch for unnecessary straining of those muscles that are supposed to be relaxed. Initially this is hard to follow nevertheless it becomes easier with some practice. This habit of differentiating between different muscles for the pressure becomes very useful in other areas of life too. It enables you to relax better while driving during rush hour. While doing normal daily tasks it makes you aware of the unnecessary tension on different parts of your body. You are watchful even while talking to someone or while brushing your teeth or when stuck in a traffic jam. You learn to ask yourself, 'Am I holding my breath, are my shoulders tense, is my neck stiff, are my fingers curled?' etc. etc. These acts are unnecessary and they dissipate energy. Yoga teaches you how to relax and gives you time free of worries and regrets, impatience and anxieties.

5) Breathing:

Monitoring your breathing is an integral part of Yoga. Common mistakes such as holding of breath or breathing deliberately occur during Yoga. Both these mistakes must be avoided. Holding back on breath gives headaches, fatigue and thus the benefits of Yoga are lost by improper or inadequate breathing.

6) Anantha Samapatti (Merging with the Infinite):
Ultimate goal of Yoga is the amalgamation of self into the greater self. Yuja means to combine or to connect. A connection of Atma and Parmatma is the merging of the body and the spirit. Yoga is a way of life. It's a total integration. According to Patanjali (founder

of Yoga), two things define Yoga postures; a stable and comfortable body posture and Anantha Samapatti. Therefore you cannot separate bodily postures from meditation. In fact a body that has become flexible and steady through practice of various positions becomes a good basis for the ultimate transcendental state of mind (Samadhi). The kriya (cleansing processes) purify the body. Mudra and bandha bring the necessary stability of mind and concentration, initially on one's breathing (pranadharana) and then on God (Ishwarpranidhana). Initially the mind wanders a lot and that's o.k. One should let it wander. Later one should count his breaths and should observe the inner and outer flow of air through the air passages. (pranadharna). This will enable him to concentrate better on himself (sakshibhavana). In the beginning it will be difficult to concentrate since the body postures are not that steady. But with practice it becomes better and better. For this one must purposely take away his mind from body posture and focus it on to the breathing process (pranadharana).

Benefits

If you follow the basic rules, several benefits can be reaped. Maintenance of body stretches makes the body supple, lean, flexible and stable. Breathing techniques purify the blood and cleanse nasal passages and sinuses. Stress relief is the greatest of all the benefits. Relaxing positions in Yoga teach you to relax your muscles and let the gravity work on your body. The ability to

140

differentiate between tension on different parts of the body, i.e. to stretch one muscle group while relaxing all the others teaches you to relax and not waste energy during your daily routine. The part about concentration is important in providing relief to your mind from worry and stress of everyday activities. Here is a detailed look at some of the major benefits of Yoga.

1. Stress relief

Stress, tension, anxiety are the inevitable features of modern day life. Yoga offers many techniques to cope up with the stress and anxiety. A stress free mind reduces the chances of catching a disease to half, this has been widely known by now. Yoga teaches very effective breathing and relaxing techniques to achieve this. Yoga also helps you to feel relaxed quicker and raise your energy reserve by teaching you how to let the gravity work on your body. Half of the fatigue in any activity comes from improper and inadequate breathing and by holding breath unnecessarily. Yoga teaches you how to breathe adequately and how not to make your body tense and stiff while doing other daily tasks too. The principle of focused stretching teaches you how to not waste energy during your daily routine. It makes you aware of the unnecessary tension on different parts of your body. Yoga teaches you to relax fully and gives you time free of worries and regrets and impatience and anxieties. People having busy schedules who are used to being in action all the time, must understand that relaxing is not a crime or not a waste of time. On the contrary it gives you new energy to do your tasks better.

2. Feeling energized and refreshed

Adequate breathing plays a great role in rejuvenating and refreshing mind and body. Breathing techniques in Yoga provide abundant supply of oxygen to the lungs, cleanse nasal passages and sinuses and thus help feel refreshed. A body that has become lean and flexible with stretches and maintenance of the stretches gets purified by breathing techniques and becomes energized. Various Yoga stretches induce a balanced secretion of hormones, which subsequently rejuvenates the whole body and one feels refreshed and energized as a result.

3. Flexibility of mind and body

Apart from the relaxing effect, yoga also consists of many body stretches which when maintained for a few minutes give a wonderful flexibility to our muscles. One starts wondering, 'Am I the same person who used to be so stiff?' In many chronic disorders of the spine, Yoga has helped many people to reduce the frequency and intensity of the disorder such as spondylitis, arthritis etc. Maintenance of body stretches makes the body supple, lean, flexible and stable. In the process, not only your body but also your mind becomes flexible. The mind acquires faith that things can change favorably given enough time.

4. Relief from chronic disorders.
Yoga is particularly good for having control over breath and spine.

Breath and spine are like wild animals. You force them to do something they pounce on you. You coax them, be patient with them, they can be tamed to any extent. Many Yoga stretches make the spine strong and flexible. Time and again Yoga has proved to be a blessing for all kinds of disorders of the back. The technique of exhaling twice longer than inhaling (Pranayama) gives abundant supply of oxygen to blood and many impurities of blood are cured. The deliberate exhaling technique (Shwasanmargshuddhi) cleanse the nasal passage and the sinuses. They help get rid of chronic sinus trouble or clogging of nasal passage for many people. That makes the lungs and respiratory organs stronger. The abdominal breathing technique (Kapalbhati) helps people with asthma or weak diaphragm to breathe easily.

5. Focus of mind
Practice of Yoga helps in getting better focus of mind. Meditation, being part of Yoga, teaches you how to focus better and achieve more from any activity. Dharana, which means narrowed focus on a subject by restricting Chitta (mind) is one of the 8 limbs of Ashtangayoga. It teaches you to get rid of all other thoughts from the mind and focus on the target. People have benefited enormously in terms of focus of mind by doing meditation (Dhyana) and Dharana throughout all ages.

6. Benefits at not-so-perfect level
Even if one cannot achieve perfection in an Asana, the benefits of

an Asana are still available at a not-so-perfect level such as calmer mind, better flexibility, better blood pressure, lower pulse rate and better endocrine function. Whatever state of Asana one is in, if one maintains the pose comfortably, body gets the necessary massage and stretch. There is a better secretion of endocrine glands as a result of the steady and sufficient stretch. The brain cells get the necessary signals and mind becomes calmer. Breath is more controlled and as a result feels refreshed. All of this happens regardless of the level of perfection. It's the steadiness and level of comfort that's more important than perfection.

Philosophy

Ashtangayoga
Among the many proponents of Yoga, Patanjali (2nd century B.C) is the most well known and most revered of all and is well accepted as the founder of Yoga. His book Shripatanjali Darshan which is a collection of hymns (also called as Patanjali's Yoga Sutras) is held in high esteem by the experts and practitioners and is known as one of the most revered reference book (a workbook for actual practice) on Yoga. Patanjali's Yoga is called Patanjala (that of Patanjali) and is also considered as Rajayoga, which means the royal Yoga or the supreme, sublime Yoga since it consists of practices that lead to spiritual liberation (Moksha). Rajayoga is a part of Sankhya philosophy and is known to awaken Kundalini (Complete opening of Chakra when reached in transcendental state of meditation) and results into complete

spiritual enlightenment if practiced regularly.

Patanjalayoga is also called Ashtangayoga since it has 8 dimensions or 8 limbs. Ashta means 8 and Anga means dimension or a limb in Sanskrit. Yama (Rules for the social life), Niyama (Rules for personal development), Asana (Yoga Posture), Pranayama (Prolonged and controlled breathing), Pratyahara (withdrawal of senses), Dharana (narrowed focusing on a subject), Dhyana (continued experience of meditation), Samadhi (transcendental state in which there is only an essence of pure existence) are the 8 limbs of Ashtangayoga. The first four dimensions make up the exoteric (Bahiranga) part of Ashtangayoga while the last four dimensions make up the esoteric (Antaranga) part of Ashtangayoga. Out of the 8 limbs of Ashtangayoga, Asana and Pranayama are the only two limbs that generally stand for the term Yoga in its most popular form.

Hathayoga
In the 15th century A.D. Yogi Swatmaram founded one of the six systems of Yoga called Hathayoga. Although the term Hatha in Sanskrit means being forceful, Hathayoga is not about Hatha but is about the balance between the two principles of the body. Ha and Tha are essentially symbols. Ha means surya (sun). Tha means chandra (moon). Right nostril (Pingala) is the Surya nadi while the left nostril (Ida) is the Chandra nadi. Just the way the sun and the moon balance the life cycle of the world; the two nostrils balance the life cycle of the body. Nadi is a channel

through which the life force flows. Hathayoga helps to maintain this balance by correcting the functional disorders of the body and bringing mental peace. Hathayogapradipika is the standard textbook on Hathayoga written by Yogi Swatmaram. Hathayoga accepts Patanjala Yoga as standard. Although it's a completely independent school of philosophy in its own right, it's essentially based upon the philosophy of Rajayoga expounded in Patanjali's Yogasutra. In fact, every school of philosophy culminates into Rajayoga since the aim of every school is the same as Rajayoga i.e. to attain ever-lasting peace and happiness.

Hathayoga consists of

a. Asana (body positions or stretches e.g. mountain pose, cobra pose)

b.   Pranayama (controlled breathing techniques e.g. Ujjayi, Anuloma Viloma)

c.   Kriya (cleansing processes e.g. Kapalbhati)

d.   Bandha and Mudra (Locks and symbol poses e.g. Udiyana bandha, Jivha bandha, Simhamudra)

As per Hathayoga, Asana, Pranayama, Kriya, Bandha and Mudra are stepping stones to achieve the ultimate psycho spiritual effect of Rajayoga. They create the necessary foundation of stable and calm mind and body for Rajayoga. There are however subtle differences between Patanjala Yoga and Hathayoga. Patanjali emphasizes more on the psycho spiritual effect of Yoga rather than the physical aspects and actual techniques of Asana and

Pranayama. His Asana and Pranayama are also much simpler and easier to do than the ones in Hathayoga. For this he recommends least amount of efforts (Prayatnay Shaithilyam) and maintaining a steady, rhythmic tempo and a stable, comfortable body position. Patanjali's Yogasutra discuss Asana and Pranayama only in the chapter of Kriyayoga (part of Sadhana pada) as the tool to achieve physical and mental health. On the other hand, the emphasis of Hathayoga is more on the techniques of Asana and Pranayama, Kriya, Bandha and Mudra.

Philosophy of Yogasutra:
Patanjali's Yogasutra consists of 195 sutra and 4 Pada (sections or chapters): Samadhi pada, Sadhana Pada, Vibhuti Pada and Kaivalya pada. Kriyayoga, the chapter on the actual practice of Yoga is a part of Sadhana Pada (section about the means of study and practice of Yoga). Kriyayoga discusses Asana and Pranayama viz. the physical part of Yoga. Just to give a glimpse of Patanjali's philosophy, here are a few thoughts from the Samadhi Pada and Sadhana Pada of Yogasutra: According to Patanjali, meaning and purpose of Yoga is to attain Samadhi (ultimate transcendental state in which there is sense of pure existence and nothing else). Yoga is a union of mind and body. It's compared with a calm river, which flows down towards its inclined bed without efforts. Thus Yoga is more than a physical exercise. To be able to concentrate your mind is the greatest benefit of Yoga. Yoga is nothing but self-study. Purpose of Yoga is to be self-aware. Yoga teaches you to be

nearer to nature and lead a healthy life. For this you need determination and faith in Yoga.

Tapaswadhyayeshwarpranidhanani Kriyayogah
Tapa (austerities), Swadhyaya (reading of scriptures), Ishwarpranidhana. Tapa is to make body alert and active glowing with health. Swadhyaya is the continuous study to sharpen the intellect. These sadhanas are to be used to wipe out faults of human nature. There are five kleshas (bad tendencies) such as avidya (ignorance), asmita (ego), Rag (attraction-affection), dwesh (hatred) and abhinivesh (self insistence, stubbornness). These five vrittis disappear by Dhyana. Yogaschittavrittinirodhah. By practice of Yoga, all the functional modifications of the mind completely cease. Control of your mind is what Yoga is about. You have to involve your mind in the Asana. Asana is an instrument to Yoga. Body postures, maintenance and rounds of an asana are to be done according to one's own capacity. Retention is more desirable than repetition. Meditation cannot be separated from Yoga. Prayatne Shaithilyam anantha samapatti. While doing Yogasana (Yogic postures), two things need to be observed. One is to be relaxed mentally and physically. The second one is Anantha samapatti. It means to merge with something infinite. Patanjali says that all good things happen when you stop trying hard. You become one with Ishwara, you let go your control and forget that you are in particular body posture. Yoga should be the way of life.

CHAPTER EIGHT

Types of Yoga

With the popularity of yoga rising throughout the western world, you have probably heard about it's healing powers by now. However, you still aren't sure exactly what kind of yoga may be right for your lifestyle. Chances are, you have probably asked everyone you know who practices yoga. While they may have a few suggestions, they may be bias in their decision making when it comes to which type of yoga you should choose. Iit is fairly simple to find the right kind of yoga for you. Especially if you have all of the information there is to know about yoga. First and foremost you should try to consider why you are planning on entering the yoga lifestyle. Whether it was suggested to you from your doctor for medical treatment, or if it is a means for you to reconnect with a healthy lifestyle. Just remember that you aren't alone. Many people struggle with trying to find the right yoga class for them. Some can spent years jumping from class to class, type to type, or different yoga teachers before finding the right match. You may find yourself drawn to the names of each yoga class, often times witty and inspiring. However, I would suggest making your decision on more than just the location or name of your yoga class. Instead taking the time to sit down with each of the teachers, and getting a feel for their technique of teaching. It may be helpful if you can find a teacher that will allow you to sit in on each type of class. This will give you a first-hand view of what would be expected of you during your yoga class. While some may promote the use of props, and focus on slow and controlled movements. Others may focus on spirituality, or exercise. All of which are beneficial to many different people in their walks of life. However, power-yoga may not be the best choice if you suffer from chronic back pain. For this reason, you should take care in choosing the right type of yoga. Before we look into the different types of classes and what you can expect you should first remember that as with any exercise program; you should first consult with your doctor. This is especially true if you have any diagnosed health problems that reduce your range of motion. Once you have begun to visit the many different yoga classes available in your area, you will find that there is a common denominator among them all. That of which is that they are focused on bringing oneness to one's life. A unity between body, mind, and soul. Regardless of the fact that this oneness is all something we hold inside of ourselves on a daily basis. However, most people will find that it can be difficult to reach this place in our own selves without a little help. Unfortunately there is no real way to answer the question of "what type of yoga is right for me?". It is more or less an moment of inspiration that you will find enter your mind once you have found the right class. As with so many things in life, yoga is specialized. However there are many different options to choose from. No one yoga class is going to be right for everyone who practices yoga. Just like no one yoga prop or work out wear will be right for one person. Think of it as a "fitting" for your lifestyle. Try your yoga class on for size, if it doesn't fit your lifestyle, your schedule, or your medical needs;

150

then you should probably try to find something different. While it is a common misconception among newcomers to yoga. You don't need to have a particular religion or belief to practice yoga. Just as you don't need to be of any one shape, or size to practice yoga. Everyone can and will benefit from the healing nature of yoga. It is even common for families to practice yoga together. If this is your plan, then finding a low-impact yoga will be imperative for younger children. Which will allow all of you to relax while getting healthy together. This of course is one of the many reasons that yoga has become so popular in the western world. As we all fight to keep our lifestyles healthy in a stressful and fast-pace lifestyle. We find that there just isn't enough time to run from one yoga class to another. Instead finding one class that will fit as a whole with your group of yoga friends, or family will help to keep your schedule relatively un-scathed. The different types of yoga can be fairly difficult to differentiate. However, there are a few key differences that can help you choose which yoga is right for you. Whether you are looking for a high-impact yoga to help you drop pounds quickly; or simply trying to find relief from arthritis, or other chronic pain. There is a yoga that will be the perfect fit for you! Hatha yoga (of which means union) is a term for yoga that employs both physical, and breathing exercise to calm the mind. This is only one of eight branches of traditional yoga, which has been passed down for generations in ancient Indian philosophy. It is thought that this style of yoga can help to attain enlightenment. Among these types of yoga that have stemmed from Hatha, you will find Raga, Mantra, and Tantra. All of which are considered to be philosophical styles of yoga, which are focused on elevating a person's mental state. It is common for Hatha yoga classes to ask their practitioners to follow a certain dietary conservation as well as ethical codes of living. There are several different disciplines that you will find practiced in Hatha yoga. However due to it's popularity, some classes may even teach a fusion of several different styles of yoga. Including Hatha yoga. Most of these hybrid yoga classes (especially those that include Hatha yoga) are often times the best for beginner yoga practitioners. Simply because they will offer a wider range of poses, breathing, and physical elements. All of which are needed to practice yoga safely and get the most out of your workout. While Hatha yoga has increased in popularity within the western world. There are many other kinds that can be found here in the United states alone. Ashtanga Viniyasa is one of the most increasingly popular forms of yoga in the last few years. It is a physical and mentally challenging form of yoga. Of which focuses on the unity between movement and breathing. However, this form of yoga can be fairly taxing and shouldn't be utilized for anyone with severe medical conditions. If you are a beginner, it is imperative to join a beginners Ashtanga class, so that you are able to learn at your own speed without posing an injury risk to yourself. Along with Hatha and Ashtanga Viniyasa yoga's you will find a few other choices to choose from. One of which being Sivananda yoga. Which is based around as little as twelve postures. One such posture sequence includes the sun salutation. Of which focuses on breathing and meditation. This is one of the most well-rounded yoga classes that can be found today. It is especially suitable for all levels of expertise, ages, and physical abilities. Making it one of the most family friendly forms of yoga available. Another popular form of yoga is Viniyoga. Of which is known for it's personalized touch. Each session of Viniyoga is tailored specially for the individual practitioner and their needs. These classes can vary from as short as fifteen minutes to two to three hours. However it is one of the best one-on-one yoga training that you can find. This is especially wonderful for anyone who might find it difficult to follow an instructor within a large class. This class is particularly well suited for children and those with medical conditions. Simply because it is so personal, and allows the trainer to keep your body, health, and physical limitations in mind when creating your routine. The last form of yoga that is commonly practiced in the western world is Iyengar. Which is a slower and more precise means of practicing yoga. It is by far the most practiced yoga throughout the world (spanning not only in the western world). It plays in important role in one's bodily alignment and posture. This is particularly well suited for those with back-pain or any other severe or chronic pain. This form of yoga is also particularly suitable for seniors, as they practice with many different props to aid in their posture progression. Remember, as with any new workout regiment that you should always know your own body's limitation. This will help you to choose the right style of yoga class for you. There is no right or wrong answer, simply knowing what you can and cannot handle is key. Regardless of the class, you should become prepared once you have chosen the right type of yoga for you. Your yoga instructor will be able to give you a list of the items you will need, whether it be yoga mats, blocks, blankets, or any other prop. It is best to come prepared!

Yoga Philosophy

Yoga is an ancient art that goes way beyond the practice of asanas - postures. It is a philosophy that goes back to the times before the religions existed more than 2,000 years ago. It is a philosophy that talks about union. It talks about union between all human beings and also about union with a greater energy that itself connects us all.

What is Yoga?
Yoga is an ancient art that has the aim of bringing the practitioner back to the true self. The ancient scriptures tell us that the true self is the state of bliss. It is a state of inner happiness. The sage Patanjali who wrote the 'Yoga Sutra' - an ancient recorded text on yoga codifying the system to date - gave the definition of yoga as 'Yoga chiti vriti nirodha'. This translates from the original Sanskrit into English to meaning that yoga is the stopping of the fluctuations of the psyche. Historically there have been two main paths of yoga -- raja yoga and hatha yoga - and these both ultimately aim for control over the mind. Asana practice - the practice of yoga postures - was created in order to stabilise us for sitting during meditation. Yoga was created ultimately to bring us into meditation and hence deeper states of awareness.

Dhyana
Now the next question arises what is meditation or dhyana in Sanskrit? Meditation is the stilling of the mind by the stilling of the body.Also pranayama - the breathing techniques of yoga - aim to still the breath and hence still the mind. Our meditational practices in yoga help us to overcome the ego. The ego is individuality. But in reality we are all connected and with yoga we realise this connection. The definition of yoga is union. Through the practice of yoga one realises the union between the you who you think you are, that is your individual consciousness, and the you who you really are - that is you are a part of a supreme consciousness. In order to transcend between the individual consciousness and the supreme consciousness one needs to overcome the ego. And in order to overcome the ego we need what the Upanishad texts describe as Vivek Chudamani. This is the crown jewel of the power of discrimination over what is real and what is not. Hence we need to be able to see that really there is no I but that we are all connected. We need to establish what it means to come back to the true self - or what is self realisation. Self realisation is in essence identifying yourself as peace and happiness. Once you have made this true identification you will just radiate peace and happiness.

The Chakras
One way of looking at yoga is in terms of the chakras (energy points within us). Now yoga aims for the ultimate functioning of all the chakras within us. This lifts us from individual

consciousness to supreme consciousness.

The Vedas
Now the Vedas - the scriptures which talk about knowledge - say that there are three defects in the mind. These are mala which is dirt, waste, excessive thoughts and emotions. Then there is vikshep which is instability and then there is avaran which means cover. The presence of avaran means that it is very hard for us to see the truth. The ancient philosophy of India was named Sanathana Dharma which can be translated as meaning the eternal law. It saw everything in the universe as being connected, as having a spiritual union - that is man, animals, nature, the whole universe. In Vedic times - the times in which the Vedas were written - the world was called Vasudevakudambakam which means one world family. When we consider the world as one family, we experience true spirituality. The world at that time was seen as being beyond the differences brought about by race, country or religion. Spirituality is about seeing the unity in all things.

The Paths of Yoga
Moving on from this knowledge, it is important for us to understand that there are several different paths of yoga all of which lead us back to self realisation or inner happiness. Karma yoga is the yoga of action. It is about removing mala. There are two different types of action or karma. Sakam involves looking for the fruit of one's actions whereas nishkam is purer. It involves not

156

looking for the fruit's of one's actions but acting through a pure heart and pure mind with no thought for expectation. Living a life of nishkam karma leads to a happier, more well balanced and peaceful life. Bhakti yoga is the yoga of devotion. There exists conditional devotion, however unconditional devotion is what is needed to remove vikshep or instability. Gyana yoga is the yoga of knowledge. It exists in order to remove avaran or cover. Gyana yoga talks a lot about the nature of consciousness. Now the nature of consciousness can be described as 'sat chit anand'. 'Sat' is existence or truth. We are all immortal in the sense that we are all souls and the soul itself is immortal. This is our true nature. We are all in search of our true immortal selves - our souls. This is why we constantly aim to live a longer life - we are trying to connect with our true selves - our immortal souls. 'Chit' is wisdom - hence we are all looking for wisdom, we are looking for the wisdom that inherently is inside every one of us. 'Anand' is bliss. Happiness is that which we have all always looked for and in the deepest core of our beings we are all essentially happiness or bliss. On the basis of sat chit anand we are all looking for self realisation or inner happiness through knowledge. Raja yoga is the kingly path. Just as a king brings law and order into his kingdom, the practitioner of raja yoga rules the kingdom within - the kingdom of the senses, so rather than being ruled by the senses, the yogi is in a state of peace and has his/her senses under control. The yogi brings law and order within.

Vedanta

After the Vedic period of Indian philosophy, the Vedantic period commenced. Vedanta means the end of the Vedas - the time where knowledge ceases and self realisation begins.Within the Vedantic tradition of philosophy, we read that there are five layers above the consciousness which stop us from identifying with who we are. We are all actually so caught up in these 5 layers that we think we are these 5 layers. These layers are known in Vedanta as the 'panch kosha'. The word 'panch' means five and the word 'kosha' means envelopes or coverings over our consciousness. With the practice of yoga we move towards the innermost layer. The first layer is called the food body or the physical body. This is known as the annamaya kosha. It is our physical body composed of the nutritients we have eaten - protein, minerals and so forth. Many times we identify ourselves with the physical body and do not look beyond that. Even when we are only looking at the physical body it is important to realise that the food we eat makes up our body and our brain. Therefore by eating healthily and also by exercising we maintain a healthy and hence happy physical and mental state. The second layer is known as the pranamaya kosha and this is the energy or etheric body. Prana can be called breath, oxygen or vital energy and relates to the chi of Chinese philosophy. Oxygen is needed for every cell of our body. Trees and plants release oxygen hence we feel alive when we are surrounded by and at one with nature. The third layer is known as the manomaya kosha or the mental body.

From this understanding we can appreciate that the mind and the body are connected. This is why we are physically more healthy when we keep a positive outlook. Laughter and happiness always create good health.

The fourth layer is the gyanamaya kosha or intuitive body. This is where we experience our sixth sense. The answers to all of our questions are found in reality in the fourth layer. And to be in the awareness of the fifth layer is our ultimate aim as yogis -- this is the bliss body - or anandmaya kosha. We experience this when we have transcended the ego completely and have become aware of who we truly are and our connection with everything. Yoga is a journey that takes us from annamaya kosha to anandmaya kosha. Once we have reached anandmaya kosha we then live in the bliss body. It can be said that meditation is a practice that allows us to go beyond the mind and senses to the deeper levels to see who we truly are.

Within the practices of yoga, asanas work on the food body, dhyana or meditation works on the mental further and further towards the deepest kosha. pranayama and works on the energy body. Hence the three practices of yoga push us.

Turiya

A 'turiya' is a person who has transcended the five koshas. The

Turiya state is the transcendental self. It is not affected by anything - neither likes nor dislikes. It is in a balanced state. When we reach this state - when we are in the bliss body - then we are beyond both pleasure and pain. We practice yoga in order to move away from being the body, the mind and the breath and just move to being the person on the inside.

The Ashtanga
The raja yoga of Patanjali talks about controlling the mind and hence the breath and hence the body. It has eight limbs attached to it - the asthanga. The word asht means eight and the word anga means limbs. The first steps of the asthanga are yama and niyama. Yama are social rules and regulations and niyama are personal rules and regulations. Just these two limbs alone are enough to give one self realisation. The other paths of yoga also take one to self realisation. To discuss these further, yama includes ahimsa (non violence), satya (truth and honesty, asteya (non stealing), bramacharya (functioning according to the supreme consciousness - which leads to acting in balance) and aparigraha (non accumulation or a sense of non possession).
Niyama includes sauch (cleanliness including mental cleanliness), santosh (contentment), tapa (austerity or self discipline), swadhyaya (self study) and Ishwar parnidhan (belief in the Supreme or seeing the Supreme in everything).

The eight limbs of yoga, the asthanga, are as follows - yama, niyama, asana, pranayama, pratyahara, dharna, dhyan and samadhi.

Dharna is one pointedness where one is so focused on the object of concentration that all other thoughts disappear. Pratyahara is withdrawal from the senses. Continuous practice of asanas and pranayama brings one to pratyahara. All the techniques of meditation are pratyahara. Samadhi is oneness with the universe. Once one has crossed dhyan and reached Samadhi, the awareness of 'I' disappears. There is only oneness with the focus of your meditation, and ultimately with the universe. At Samadhi the ego disappears and there is a realisation that we are all connected. Within Samadhi there is savikalpa samadhi where some seeds of 'I' are left and there is nirvikalpa samadhi where no seeds are left. In yoga the aim is to move towards nirvikalpa samadhi.

Kewalya
According to Patanjali the ultimate aim of yoga is towards kewalya where there is no return from samadhi. This is the state of oneness with the universe in which there is no sense of self, no sense of 'I', no ego and no awareness of it to return to. It is just a state where we realise how we are all connected and it is a state of bliss because it is where we have overcome all the attachments of the pleasures and pains that attachment to this material world brings. It is where we connect with the supreme self and experience our natural state of bliss. It is at this point where we have realised our true self through the practice of yoga. Yoga goes beyond the mere practice of asanas, beyond even meditation and pranayama and in fact brings us closer to our original state of self

realisation. Shanti. Yoga teaches us to go deeper within ourselves and in this deeper awareness there is a great sense of shanti or peace we can all draw from. Ultimately as good yoga students it is this sense of peace within which we are all searching for. Yoga is an ancient art that goes way beyond the practice of asanas - postures. It is a philosophy that goes back to the times before the religions existed more than 2,000 years ago. It is a philosophy that talks about union. It talks about union between all human beings and also about union with a greater energy that itself connects us all.

What is Yoga?

Yoga is an ancient art that has the aim of bringing the practitioner back to the true self. The ancient scriptures tell us that the true self is the state of bliss. It is a state of inner happiness. The sage Patanjali who wrote the 'Yoga Sutra' - an ancient recorded text on yoga codifying the system to date - gave the definition of yoga as 'Yoga chiti vriti nirodha'. This translates from the original Sanskrit into English to meaning that yoga is the stopping of the fluctuations of the psyche. Historically there have been two main paths of yoga -- raja yoga and hatha yoga - and these both ultimately aim for control over the mind. Asana practice - the practice of yoga postures - was created in order to stabilise us for sitting during meditation. Yoga was created ultimately to bring us into meditation and hence deeper states of awareness.

Dhyana

Now the next question arises what is meditation or dhyana in Sanskrit? Meditation is the stilling of the mind by the stilling of the body. Also pranayama - the breathing techniques of yoga - aim to still the breath and hence still the mind. Our meditational practices in yoga help us to overcome the ego. The ego is individuality. But in reality we are all connected and with yoga we realise this connection. The definition of yoga is union. Through the practice of yoga one realises the union between the you who you think you are, that is your individual consciousness, and the you who you really are - that is you are a part of a supreme consciousness. In order to transcend between the individual consciousness and the supreme consciousness one needs to overcome the ego. And in order to overcome the ego we need what the Upanishad texts describe as Vivek Chudamani. This is the crown jewel of the power of discrimination over what is real and what is not. Hence we need to be able to see that really there is no I but that we are all connected.

We need to establish what it means to come back to the true self - or what is self realisation. Self realisation is in essence identifying yourself as peace and happiness. Once you have made this true identification you will just radiate peace and happiness.

The Chakras

One way of looking at yoga is in terms of the chakras (energy points within us). Now yoga aims for the ultimate functioning of all the chakras within us. This lifts us from individual consciousness to supreme consciousness.

The Vedas
Now the Vedas - the scriptures which talk about knowledge - say that there are three defects in the mind. These are mala which is dirt, waste, excessive thoughts and emotions. Then there is vikshep which is instability and then there is avaran which means cover. The presence of avaran means that it is very hard for us to see the truth. The ancient philosophy of India was named Sanathana Dharma which can be translated as meaning the eternal law. It saw everything in the universe as being connected, as having a spiritual union - that is man, animals, nature, the whole universe. In Vedic times - the times in which the Vedas were written - the world was called Vasudevakudambakam which means one world family. When we consider the world as one family, we experience true spirituality. The world at that time was seen as being beyond the differences brought about by race, country or religion. Spirituality is about seeing the unity in all things.

The Paths of Yoga
Moving on from this knowledge, it is important for us to understand that there are several different paths of yoga all of which lead us back to self realisation or inner happiness. Karma yoga is the yoga of action. It is about removing mala. There are two different types of action or karma. Sakam involves looking for the fruit of one's actions whereas nishkam is purer. It involves not

looking for the fruit's of one's actions but acting through a pure heart and pure mind with no thought for expectation. Living a life of nishkam karma leads to a happier, more well balanced and peaceful life. Bhakti yoga is the yoga of devotion. There exists conditional devotion, however unconditional devotion is what is needed to remove vikshep or instability. Gyana yoga is the yoga of knowledge. It exists in order to remove avaran or cover. Gyana yoga talks a lot about the nature of consciousness. Now the nature of consciousness can be described as 'sat chit anand'. 'Sat' is existence or truth. We are all immortal in the sense that we are all souls and the soul itself is immortal. This is our true nature. We are all in search of our true immortal selves - our souls. This is why we constantly aim to live a longer life - we are trying to connect with our true selves - our immortal souls. 'Chit' is wisdom - hence we are all looking for wisdom, we are looking for the wisdom that inherently is inside every one of us. 'Anand' is bliss. Happiness is that which we have all always looked for and in the deepest core of our beings we are all essentially happiness or bliss. On the basis of sat chit anand we are all looking for self realisation or inner happiness through knowledge. Raja yoga is the kingly path. Just as a king brings law and order into his kingdom, the practitioner of raja yoga rules the kingdom within - the kingdom of the senses, so rather than being ruled by the senses, the yogi is in a state of peace and has his/her senses under control. The yogi brings law and order within.

Vedanta
After the Vedic period of Indian philosophy, the Vedantic period

commenced. Vedanta means the end of the Vedas - the time where knowledge ceases and self realisation begins. Within the Vedantic tradition of philosophy, we read that there are five layers above the consciousness which stop us from identifying with who we are. We are all actually so caught up in these 5 layers that we think we are these 5 layers. These layers are known in Vedanta as the 'panch kosha'. The word 'panch' means five and the word 'kosha' means envelopes or coverings over our consciousness. With the practice of yoga we move towards the innermost layer.

The first layer is called the food body or the physical body. This is known as the annamaya kosha. It is our physical body composed of the nutritients we have eaten - protein, minerals and so forth. Many times we identify ourselves with the physical body and do not look beyond that. Even when we are only looking at the physical body it is important to realise that the food we eat makes up our body and our brain. Therefore by eating healthily and also by exercising we maintain a healthy and hence happy physical and mental state.

The second layer is known as the pranamaya kosha and this is the energy or etheric body. Prana can be called breath, oxygen or vital energy and relates to the chi of Chinese philosophy. Oxygen is needed for every cell of our body. Trees and plants release oxygen hence we feel alive when we are surrounded by and at one with nature.

The third layer is known as the manomaya kosha or the mental body. From this understanding we can appreciate that the mind and the body are connected. This is why we are physically more healthy when we keep a positive outlook. Laughter and happiness always create good health.

The fourth layer is the gyanamaya kosha or intuitive body. This is where we experience our sixth sense. The answers to all of our ⬚uestions are found in reality in the fourth layer.

And to be in the awareness of the fifth layer is our ultimate aim as yogis -- this is the bliss body - or anandmaya kosha. We experience this when we have transcended the ego completely and have become aware of who we truly are and our connection with everything. Yoga is a journey that takes us from annamaya kosha to anandmaya kosha. Once we have reached anandmaya kosha we then live in the bliss body.

It can be said that meditation is a practice that allows us to go beyond the mind and senses to the deeper levels to see who we truly are. Within the practices of yoga, asanas work on the food body, pranayama works on the energy body and dhyana or meditation works on the mental body. Hence the three practices of yoga push us further and further towards the deepest kosha.

Turiya

A 'turiya' is a person who has transcended the five koshas. The Turiya state is the transcendental self. It is not affected by anything - neither likes nor dislikes. It is in a balanced state. When we reach this state - when we are in the bliss body - then we are beyond both pleasure and pain. We practice yoga in order to move away from being the body, the mind and the breath and just move to being the person on the inside.

The Ashtanga

The raja yoga of Patanjali talks about controlling the mind and hence the breath and hence the body. It has eight limbs attached to it - the asthanga. The word asht means eight and the word anga means limbs. The first steps of the asthanga are yama and niyama. Yama are social rules and regulations and niyama are personal rules and regulations. Just these two limbs alone are enough to give one self realisation. The other paths of yoga also take one to self realisation. To discuss these further, yama includes ahimsa (non violence), satya (truth and honesty, asteya (non stealing), bramacharya (functioning according to the supreme consciousness - which leads to acting in balance) and aparigraha (non accumulation or a sense of non possession).

Niyama includes sauch (cleanliness including mental cleanliness), santosh (contentment), tapa (austerity or self discipline), swadhyaya (self study) and Ishwar parnidhan (belief in the Supreme or seeing the Supreme in everything). The eight limbs of yoga, the asthanga, are as follows - yama, niyama, asana, pranayama, pratyahara, dharna, dhyan and samadhi. Dharna is one pointedness where one is so focused on the object of concentration that all other thoughts disappear.

Pratyahara is withdrawal from the senses. Continuous practice of asanas and pranayama brings one to pratyahara. All the techniques of meditation are pratyahara.

Samadhi is oneness with the universe. Once one has crossed

dhyan and reached Samadhi, the awareness of 'I' disappears. There is only oneness with the focus of your meditation, and ultimately with the universe. At Samadhi the ego disappears and there is a realisation that we are all connected. Within Samadhi there is savikalpa samadhi where some seeds of 'I' are left and there is nirvikalpa samadhi where no seeds are left. In yoga the aim is to move towards nirvikalpa samadhi.

Kewalya
According to Patanjali the ultimate aim of yoga is towards kewalya where there is no return from samadhi. This is the state of oneness with the universe in which there is no sense of self, no sense of 'I', no ego and no awareness of it to return to. It is just a state where we realise how we are all connected and it is a state of bliss because it is where we have overcome all the attachments of the pleasures and pains that attachment to this material world brings. It is where we connect with the supreme self and experience our natural state of bliss. It is at this point where we have realised our true self through the practice of yoga.

Yoga goes beyond the mere practice of asanas, beyond even meditation and pranayama and in fact brings us closer to our original state of self realisation.

Shanti
Yoga teaches us to go deeper within ourselves and in this deeper awareness there is a great sense of shanti or peace we can all draw from. Ultimately as good yoga students it is this sense of peace within which we are all searching for.

Not Just Fitness

Over the past few decades, a very common misconception has taken root in the minds of people. There is a belief that Yoga, is all about fitness and exercise. An added misconception is that Yogasanas (or Asanas) are simply body movements and poses that are complex to perform but make the body supple. Yes, asana or postures do make the body supple. Just like stretching and other forms of body movements do. But Yoga and yogasanas are so much more than just fitness tricks. In the West, somewhere around the 19th Century and 20th Century, Yoga was introduced by Indians to the people, so that they too may benefit from it. As expected it was a great success. But there began a commercialization of yoga, in order to make it more appealing to the public. Yoga went from being an art, to a training session. This is something we need to understand, is extremely dangerous. Yoga isn't something that should be performed with the wrong ideas or intentions. It has consequences of its own. Yoga is a way of life. It is not a ritual to be performed, it is a habit that one makes a part of life. The ultimate aim of Yoga is to achieve liberation or Moksha. But yoga has a huge impact on our day-to-day lives.

Five basic principles of Yoga

- Asana (postures)

- Pranayama (Breathing control)

- Shavasana (Relaxation)

- Sattvic (Right Diet)

- Dhyana (Meditation)

It is only when these 5 basic principles are followed that one can call himself a practitioner of Yoga. When a person performs yoga, he surrenders himself to the universe and becomes one with the universal energy. It is a very potent source of life and should not be treated lightly.

Let us now look at some more important facets of yoga.

Schools of Yoga

In Hinduism, there are the following types of Yoga, which are to be practiced. Please note, here Yoga doesn't talk about postures. Yoga is in fact a practice. As I mentioned earlier, it is a way of life. These schools of yoga were thus, part of life.

1. Jnana Yoga
Jnana means 'knowledge' in Sanskrit. In the ancient times, when there was a system of 'Gurukul' (students stayed with teachers and gained knowledge), this was the initiation of the student into education and the realm of knowledge. The teachings included information about everything under the sun. This Jnana yoga became the foundation for yogic understanding and knowledge.

2. Bhakti Yoga
Bhakti or devotion, is an essential aspect of yoga. Through this

form of yoga, one expressed love and devotion towards God. Here God is the Supreme Being. It does not refer to any symbolic God, simply universal energy. The idea was to move the yogi, towards spiritual awakening.

3. Karma Yoga

Karma means Duty in Sanskrit. In the Hindu religion, the importance of performing ones duty or Karma, was of the highest importance. Disciplined actions and all duties had to be performed with great reverence. It is said to be the most effective way to progress in spiritual life.

4. Laya Yoga or Kundalini Yoga

It is the form of yoga performed by way of regular practice of meditation, pranayama, chanting mantra and yoga asana. It is called the yoga of awakening. One becomes aware of oneself and more conscious of the surrounding. It focuses on compassion to others and healing of the body, mind and soul.

5. Hatha Yoga

It is a system of physical techniques supplementary to a broad conception of yoga. There is a belief that Lord Shiva himself was the creator of Hatha Yoga.

This school of yoga is what deals with physical exercise and asana or postures. Hatha yoga is more known as a physical exercise in the world.

Benefits of Yoga

Yoga has physical benefits, is something which is common knowledge. But the real power of yoga is seen through its benefits on the mental and other aspects of human life.
Following are some of the major benefits of yoga.

* Perfects your posture

Yoga helps make you stand up straighter and walk taller. The whole slumped shoulder problem goes away. Also, it makes you look far more graceful and toned.

• Control of emotions

Yoga helps the body relax, which in turn helps you control your emotions. Very often, an excess of anger or any negative emotion, gets directed towards the wrong person. This happens when we can't really control our thoughts and emotions. Yoga helps to control our mind and also makes us patient.

* Makes you happier

Practising yoga, even simple breathing exercises or pranayama, helps to pump more endorphins and dopamine into the system. These are some hormones that make you feel happier. The more yoga you practice, the higher your chances of feeling happy and uplifted.

• Helps you focus

Whenever you find yourself incapable of focusing, try practicing yoga and meditation. Meditation makes you concentrate and brings to you an increased observation power.

• Improves Balance

What yogasanas do mainly, is that they direct your body's energy in a particular direction.

Practicing yoga and doing the correct postures, helps direct more energy into various directions.

This helps improve your balance.

• Relaxes muscles

If you are someone prone to muscle tension or pulling of muscles (hamstring, shoulder, etc.) then yoga can help make your body supple. Your flexibility naturally improves and you can do more activities with ease.

There are many more medical benefits too. However, there are few tested proofs that can be stated. For example, people suffering from asthma and bronchitis, are told to practice pranayama as it helps to control their breathing, which improves lung capacity. These are tested facts. But there is no evidence to suggest that Yoga can cure terminal diseases or act as a pain reliever. So we must get the facts before following any practice. Another essential point to bear in mind is that Yoga, should only be performed, after attaining some initial training from a yoga guru or instructor. This is because we may try to do some postures and end up causing serious injuries, if they aren't done appropriately. Lastly, it is always best to read books and other resources that can clearly define what Yoga really is, before going and enrolling for a class. If you have some knowledge to begin with, you will feel a lot more connected to the activity itself.

Yoga Body, and Spirit: Can We Have Both?

It's easy to understand why John Friend highly recommends the book Yoga Body: The Origins of Modern Posture Yoga "for all sincere students of yoga." Because, Mark Singleton's thesis is a well researched expose of how modern hatha yoga, or "posture practice," as he terms it, has changed within and after the practice left India. But the book is mainly about how yoga transformed in India itself in the last 150 years. How yoga's main, modern proponents-T. Krishnamacharya and his students, K. Patttabhi Jois and B. K. S. Iyengar-mixed their homegrown hatha yoga practices with European gymnastics. This was how many Indian yogis coped with modernity: Rather than remaining in the caves of the Himalayas, they moved to the city and embraced the oncoming European cultural trends. They especially embraced its more "esoteric forms of gymnastics," including the influential Swedish techniques of Ling (1766-1839). Singleton uses the word yoga as a homonym to explain the main goal of his thesis. That is, he emphasizes that the word yoga has multiple meanings, depending on who uses the term.

This emphasis is in itself a worthy enterprise for students of everything yoga; to comprehend and accept that your yoga may not be the same kind of yoga as my yoga. Simply, that there are many paths of yoga. In that regard, John Friend is absolutely right: this is by far the most comprehensive study of the culture and history of the influential yoga lineage that runs from T. Krishnamacharya's humid and hot palace studio in Mysore to Bikram's artificially heated studio in Hollywood. Singleton's study on "postural yoga" makes up the bulk of the book. But he also devotes some pages to outline the history of "traditional" yoga, from Patanjali to the Shaiva Tantrics who, based on much earlier yoga traditions, compiled the hatha yoga tradition in the middle ages and penned the famous yoga text books the Hatha Yoga Pradipika and the Geranda Samhita. It is while doing these examinations that Singleton gets into water much hotter than a Bikram sweat. Thus I hesitate in giving Singleton a straight A for his otherwise excellent dissertation. Singleton claims his project is solely the study of modern posture yoga. If he had stuck to that project alone, his book would have been great and received only accolades. But unfortunately, he commits the same blunder so many modern hatha yogis do. All yoga styles are fine, these hatha yogis say. All homonyms are equally good and valid, they claim. Except that homonym, which the cultural relativist hatha yogis perceive as an arrogant version of yoga. Why? Because its adherents, the traditionalists, claim it is a deeper, more spiritual and traditional from of yoga. This kind of ranking, thinks Singleton, is counterproductive and a waste of time.

Georg Feuerstein disagrees. Undoubtedly the most prolific and well-respected yoga scholar outside India today, he is one of those traditionalists who holds yoga to be an integral practice-a body, mind, spirit practice. So how does Feuerstein's integral yoga homonym differ from the non-integral modern posture yoga homonym presented to us by Singleton? Simply put, Feuerstein's remarkable writings on yoga have focused on the holistic practice of yoga. On the whole shebang of practices that traditional yoga developed over the past 5000 plus years: asanas, pranayama (breathing exercises), chakra (subtle energy centers), kundalini (spiritual energy), bandhas (advanced body locks), mantras, mudras (hand gestures), etc. Hence, while posture yoga primarily focuses on the physical body, on doing postures, integral yoga includes both the physical and the subtle body and involves a whole plethora of physical, mental and spiritual practices hardly ever practiced in any of today's modern yoga studios. would not have bothered to bring all this up had it not been for the fact that Singleton mentioned Feuerstein in a critical light in his book's "Concluding Reflections." In other words, it is strategically important for Singleton to critique Feuerstein's interpretation of yoga, a form of yoga which happens to pretty much coincide with my own. Singleton writes: "For some, such as best-selling yoga scholar Georg Feuerstein, the modern fascination with postural yoga can only be a perversion of the authentic yoga of tradition." Then Singleton quotes Feuerstein, who writes that when yoga reached Western shores it "was gradually stripped of its spiritual orientation and remodeled into fitness training." Singleton then correctly points out that yoga had already started this fitness change in India. He also correctly points out that fitness yoga is not apposed to any "spiritual" enterprise of yoga. But that is not exactly Feuerstein's point: he simply points out how the physical exercise part of modern yoga lacks a deep "spiritual orientation." And that is a crucial difference. Then Singleton exclaims that Feuerstein's assertions misses the "deeply spiritual orientation of some modern bodybuilding and women's fitness training in the harmonial gymnastics tradition." While I think I am quite clear about what Feuerstein means by "deeply spiritual," I am still not sure what Singleton means by it from just reading Yoga Body. And that makes an intelligent comparison difficult. Hence why did Singleton bring this up in his concluding arguments in a book devoted to physical postures? Surely to make a point.

Since he did make a point about it, I would like to respond.
According to Feuerstein, the goal of yoga is enlightenment (Samadhi), not physical fitness, not even spiritual physical fitness. Not a better, slimmer physique, but a better chance at spiritual liberation. For him, yoga is primarily a spiritual practice involving deep postures, deep study and deep meditation. Even though postures are an integral part of traditional yoga, enlightenment is possible even without the practice of posture yoga, indisputably proven by such sages as Ananda Mai Ma, Ramana Maharishi, Nisargadatta Maharaj, and others. The broader question about the goal of yoga, from the point of view of traditional yoga is this: is it possible to attain enlightenment through the practice of fitness yoga alone? The answer: Not very easy. Not even likely.

Not even by practicing the kind of fitness yoga Singleton claims is "spiritual." According to integral yoga, the body is the first and outer layer of the mind. Enlightenment, however, takes place in and beyond the fifth and innermost layer of the subtle body, or kosa, not in the physical body. Hence, from this particular perspective of yoga, fitness yoga has certain limits, simply because it cannot alone deliver the desired results. Similarily, Feuerstein and all us other traditionalists (oh, those darn labels!) are simply saying that if your goal is enlightenment, then fitness yoga probably won't do the trick. You can stand on your head and do power yoga from dawn to midnight, but you still won't be enlightened. Hence, they designed sitting yoga postures (padmasana, siddhasana, viirasana, etc) for such particular purposes. Indeed, they spent more time sitting still in meditation over moving about doing postures, as it was the sitting practices which induced the desired trance states of enlightenment, or Samadhi. In other words, you can be enlightened without ever practicing the varied hatha postures, but you probably won't get enlightened by just practicing these postures alone, no matter how "spiritual" those postures are. These are the kinds of layered insights and perspectives I sorely missed while reading Yoga Body. Hence his criticism of Feuerstein seems rather shallow and kneejerk. Singleton's sole focus on describing the physical practice and history of modern yoga is comprehensive, probably quite accurate, and rather impressive, but his insistence that there are "deeply spiritual" aspects of modern gymnastics and posture yoga misses an important point about yoga. Namely, that our bodies are only as spiritual as we are, from that space in our hearts, deep within and beyond the body. Yoga Body thus misses a crucial point many of us have the right to claim, and without having to be criticized for being arrogant or mean-minded: that yoga is primarily a holistic practice, in which the physical body is seen as the first layer of a series of ascending and all-embracing layers of being-from body to mind to spirit. And that ultimately, even the body is the dwelling place of Spirit. In sum, the body is the sacred temple of Spirit. And where does this yoga perspective hail from? According to Feuerstein, "It underlies the entire Tantric tradition, notably the schools of hatha yoga, which are an offshoot of Tantrism." In Tantra it is clearly understood that the human being is a three-tiered being-physical, mental and spiritual. Hence, the Tantrics very skillfully and carefully developed practices for all three levels of being. From this ancient perspective, it is very gratifying to see how the more spiritual, all-embracing tantric and yogic practices such as hatha yoga, mantra meditation, breathing exercises, ayurveda, kirtan, and scriptural study are increasingly becoming integral features of many modern yoga studios. So, to answer the question in the title of this article. Can we have both a limber physique and a sacred spirit while practicing yoga? Yes, of course we can. Yoga is not either/or. Yoga is yes/and. The more holistic our yoga practice becomes-that is, the more spiritual practice is added to our posture practice-the more these two seemingly opposite poles-the body and the spirit-will blend and unify. Unity was, after all, the goal of ancient Tantra. Perhaps soon someone will write a book about this new, ever-growing homonym of global yoga? Mark Singleton's Yoga Body is not such a book. But a book about this, shall we call it, neo-traditional, or holistic form of yoga would certainly be an interesting cultural exploration.

CHAPTER NINE

The Types

The term "yoga" is applied to an assortment of practices and methods that also include Hindu, Jain and Buddhist practices. In Hinduism these practices include Jnana Yoga, Bhakti Yoga, Laya Yoga and Hatha Yoga.

Ashtanga Yoga
Yoga Sutras of Pantajali, which are the oldest known written compilation about yoga, include the Raja Yoga or the Ashtanga Yoga, (the eight limbs to be practiced to attain Samadhi). The ultimate aim of the yoga practice is to obtain Samadhi or unity of the individual self with the Supreme Being. Patanjali states that one can achieve this supreme union by elimination the 'vruttis' or the different modifications of the mind. The mind can in turn be controlled by right discipline and training of the body. The Yoga-Sutra of Patanjali comprise of:

Yama: Social restraints or ethical values for living. They include: Ahimsa (Non-violence), Satya (truthfulness) Asteya (non-stealing), Brahmacharya (celibacy, fidelity to one's partner) and Aparigraha (non-possessiveness).

Niyama - They include the personal observances of - Sauca (clarity of mind, speech and body), Santosha (contentment), Tapas (perseverance). Svadhyaya (study of self, self-reflection, study of Vedas), and Ishvara-Pranidhana (contemplation of God/Supreme Being/True Self)

Asana: Literally means "seat", and in Patanjali's Sutras refers to the seated position used for meditation.

Pranayama -Prana, breath, "ayama", to restrain or stop i.e., regulation of breath

Pratyahara - Withdrawal of the sense in preparation to meditation.

Dharana - Concentration

Dhyana - Meditation.

Samadhi - Liberating one's body to attain ecstasy.Moreover, Patanjali has identified some basic obstacles that do not allow the mind from practicing yoga. He has divided them into 2 classes:

Antarayas (intruders in the path of yoga)

Viksepasahabhuvah (co-existing with mental distraction)

There are 9 Antarayas:

Vyadhi (physical illness) - If a body is suffering from some disease, it needs to be cured and restored to a healthy state. Disease causes disorder of the mind and makes it difficult to practice yoga or any other form of physical discipline

Styana (mental laziness) - The human desire to reap the fruits of action without any effort is not conducive to mental health. Strong will power needs to be employed to do away with this ailment.

Samshaya (doubt) - Faith is the only cure to dispel all arising doubts.

Pramada (heedlessness) - If one is oblivious to cultivate virtues, Yoga cannot be practiced.

Alasya (physical laziness) - Involving in healthy activities helps overcome this laziness

Avirati (detachment) - The mind needs to be detached from material objects to attain Yoga

Bhrantidarsana (false perception) - leads to self-conceit and needs to be kept away.

Alabdha- bhumikatva (non-attainment of yogic states) - Recognizing the evil traits in our personality and banishing them would help in the long run

Anavasthitatva (falling away from yogic states attained)

There are 4 Viksepasahabhuvah

Dukha - sorrow and suffering inflicting the human mind.

Daurmanasya - disappointment due to non-fulfillment of desires and ambition.

Angamejayatva - restlessness of the limbs due to mental agitation.

Shvasa and prashvasa - forced inhalation and exhalation. Controlled breathing or a balance in breathing exerts a calming influence in the mind.

Patanjali states that these impediments can be removed through meditation and devotion to God; which will pave the way for self-realization.

Vashishta Yoga:
Yoga Vashishta is supposed to have been disclosed by the Vedic sage, Vashishta to his royal disciple Lord Rama, who is said to be a reincarnation of Lord Vishnu. Yoga Vashishta comprises of 32000 shlokas. In this scripture, sage Vashishta explains the teachings of Vedanta in form of stories to Lord Rama. He teaches him about the deceptive nature of the world, teaches him the best means to attain wisdom and happiness thus showing him the path leading to the supreme spirit.

Kundalini Yoga (Laya Yoga):
This form of yoga was first introduced in The Yoga- Kundalini Upanishad in the first half of 17th century. Kundalini yoga is the yoga of consciousness. Kundalini is primal energy or Shakti, which lies dormant and is coiled at the base of the spine like a serpent. It is the energy of consciousness and awareness in any human form. Kundalini yoga is supposed to awaken the sleeping Kundalini Shakti from its coiled position at the spinal base through a series of 6 chakras, and penetrate the 7th chakra, or the crown. The purpose of this form of yoga through daily practice of kriyas and meditation in sadhana is said to be a practical technology of human consciousness to achieve their ultimate creative potential. Practicing this Kundalini Yoga regularly, leads one to be liberated from one's Karma and to realize their purpose in life (Dharma).

Nada Yoga:

The basic theory behind Nada Yoga is that the entire universe and all its inhabitants consist of sound vibrations or nadas (Sanskrit, 'nad' means sound). 'Nada' resonates to the sound of 'Om', which is the primitive form of energy. Nada yoga practices forms of exercise summoning the union of the self with God, through sound or music. The N?da yoga system divides sound or music into two categories: internal sound, anahata, and external sound, ahata. In Nada yoga, the person focuses his attention on the 'anahata' nada or the inner sound. The focus is to be primarily on the sound that is produced within the human body and not on any external vibrations. The aspirant experiences a feeling of stillness, which infuses a capacity to reconnect with the soul or the 'atman'. Nada yoga assists in tuning ourselves to all the sounds, ultimately immersing oneself with the cosmic sound, 'Om'. Yoga Sutras of Patanjali states that, the mantra 'Om' is "the sound that expresses the Supreme Being, which should be repeatedly chanted while at the same time absorbing its meaning."

Jnana yoga:

Jnana (wisdom or knowledge) is the most difficult path to achieve in Yoga and re?uires great strength of will and intellect. The primary goal of this form of yoga is to become liberated from the deceptive world of maya (thoughts and perceptions) and to achieve union of the inner Self (Atman) with the oneness of all life (Brahman). This is achieved by continuously practicing the mental techniques of self-questioning, contemplation and conscious illumination stated in the sadhana chatushtaya (Four Pillars of Knowledge). These Four Pillars are the steps toward achieving liberation. Continuous practice of these steps would cultivate spiritual insight, understanding and reduce suffering and dissatisfaction in life. The 4 steps are:

Viveka (discernment, discrimination) - deliberate intellectual effort to differentiate between the permanent and the temporary and Self and not-Self

Vairagya (detachment) - The mind needs to be detached from material objects to attain Yoga

Shatsampat (six virtues) - six mental practices of calmness, restraint, renunciation, endurance, trust and focus to stabilize the mind and emotions

Mumukshutva (yearning) - passionate desire for liberation from suffering. It is equally important to practice humility and compassion on the path of self-realization.

Bhakti Yoga:
Bhakti (devotion or love) Yoga is one of the four main paths to attain enlightenment. This form of yoga endeavors to unite the bhakta (aspirant) with the Divine. Bhakti Yoga is said to be the easiest and the most direct method to experience the unity of mind, body and spirit. Bhakti Yoga requires only an open, loving

heart, whereas Hatha Yoga requires a strong and flexible body, Raja Yoga requires a disciplined and concentrated mind, and Jnana Yoga requires a keen intellect. Bhakti Yoga complements other paths of yoga well, and it is said that jnana (knowledge or wisdom) will emerge when you immerse yourself in the devotional practices of Bhakti Yoga.

Hatha yoga
Hatha (Ha-sun; tha- moon) yoga refers to balancing the masculine aspects-active, hot, sun-and feminine aspects-receptive, cool, moon-within all of us. It creates a path toward balance and uniting the opposite forces. It strives to attain the union of mind and body by a series of asanas (postures) and pranayama (breathing exercises) as described in ancient Hindu texts. These practices help activate the Kundalini energy and purify the body of negative thoughts. It is very popular form of Yoga in the Western world currently.

Physical and Mental Wellness

The meaning of Yoga is to connect the Soul with God. Moksha (Salvation), freedom from all types of pain by living a balanced life is the ultimate goal of Yoga. Doing away with mundane and trivial desires arising in the mind is Yoga.Yoga is a technique through which man exercised control over his physical and mental being, to attain hitherto unachieved states of bliss and to be able to conjecture on God or The Supreme Soul, the Parmatma, and to dwell upon the creation and existence of this world. Yoga offers a path to final Salvation as well as a more temporal kind, temporal in terms of relieving unhappiness, the kind that certainly results from poor health. The practice or process of Yoga are very beneficial for the maintenance of health. It helps to maintain both physical and mental health, which cannot be done by either taking pills or drinking potions. Yoga helps one overcome mental depression as well as attain equilibrium between body and soul. It increases the capacity to work and benefits the brain by increasing retention power and memory.Yoga is known as Astanga or eight-faceted Yoga and these eight facets are Yama, Niyama, Asana, Pranayama, Pratyahara, Dharana, Dhyana, and Samadhi.

Yama: It stands for Ahimsa, benevolence to all living beings, respect and tolerance and objectivity in all feeling, doing and observing.

Satya (Truth): One must always speak and think truthfully.

Asteya (Abstaining from Stealing): One who overcomes such act is showered with precious stones.

Brahmacharya (Celibacy): It is when the mind fuses with the Parabrahma or the highest level of consciousness. Brahmacharya would include doing away with: thinking about sexual partners, singing about attractions, about ladies, meeting, interacting with other potential partners, other ladies, coitus and voyeurism, viewing entertainment with titillating content, reading books or discussing or viewing material with pornographic content, and Kriya Nispathi.

Rutu Kala: One must not indulge physically with any other than one's lawfully wedded wife or husband and that too only during Rutu Kala, the period which starts on the fourth day after menstruation and ends on the sixteenth.

Aparigraha: Although enjoyable, many things we do and are addicted to, such as some of the foods that we eat, are not good for us and must be given up.

Niyama: It encompasses the five concepts of Cleanliness, Contentment, Penance, Swadhyaya and Ishwari Pranidhana.

Santoshadanuttama Sukha Labha; to be truly happy and contented is a state of mind.

Vidhinoktera Margena Kricchra Chandra Yanadibhi:|

Sareera Soshanam Prahu Stapa Sasta Pa Uttanam||

This advocates leading an austere life.

Karyendrisiddhirasuddhi Kshaya Staasa:|

Practice the Vedas and Mantras of which the Gayatri Mantra is the root, strictly in accordance to the procedure prescribed in the Shastras.

Kamatos Kamatospi Yatkaromisubhasubhi|

Tatsarvam Twayivinyasya Twatparata Yuktaha karomyoham||

One should devote one's soul to God and dedicate one's work to Him regardless of whether one's work brings any material gains.

Samadhi Siddhirswareeswara Pranidhanath|

By practicing Yama and Niyama and the Asanas of Yoga, one is able to gain control of one's body, mind and soul, and thereby gain control over disease. When the focus of practice is on the Antaratma, the inner spirit of the soul, it is called Hathayoga, and when this focus is on the Atma or one's own mentality, it is called Rajayoga. To sum up, the Yoga Asanas help to condition the body, the mind and the soul so that one can overcome impervious to disease, but before Asanas may be practice, a suitable state of mental readiness must be achieved. The practice of Yoga involves the imposition of considerable self-discipline in one's diet and in the activities one pursues. A Satvic diet is advocated for those who wish to take up Yoga as a practice. The practitioner's diet must consist of foods that are healthy and provide strength and well-being, foods of the quality comparable to those that are offered to Gods. Yoga may be practiced at various levels, and so, it is a beneficial activity. The place for practicing Yogasanas must be clean and airy but not windy. It should not be performed in an unclean or offensive smell area and also never on the roof or in a basement. Before the conclusion of the session, the practitioner should have work up a light sweat. At this stage, he or she should rub down the perspiration on the body itself before bathing. At the conclusion of a session of Yogasanas, the body should not be exposed to breeze for at least an hour, otherwise it will sap strength. Perspiration should be rubbed down on the body itself, before a bath in tepid or hot water. One should not be on a fast or without nourishment when practicing Yoga. Yoga practitioners should respect and obey God, their elders, the Gurus and parents. The practice of Yoga is beneficial for all ages and genders, from the time when a child is about eight years old. Practice of Yoga is not advised for pregnant women. Regular practice of Yogasanas rejuvenates the body. It gives relief to ailments of both the body and the mind.

Asanas in Yoga and their Benefits:

The Sun Salutation (Surya Namaskara):

A proper starting point for the practice of Yoga is the Surya Namaskara or a salutation to the sun. The Sun Salutation provides happiness to the body, the mind and the senses. It is good for the heart. The regular performer will live long, be hale and hearty, with a strong and a sturdy body and keen intellect.

Kurmasana:

This exercise will reduce the formation of phlegm in the chest and throat. It is also beneficial for the heart, lungs and the cardiovascular system, besides strengthening the chest and the back.

Padmasana:

It improves the consciousness and the intellect, and brings about mental stability. On the physical level, it will reduce the fat in the thighs.

Sarvangasana:

This exercise stimulates the thyroid glands and the genitalia of both males and females. It is also useful in conditions of haemorrhoids, hernias and menstrual disorder. But it is not to be practiced by people suffering from cervical spondylitis.

Matsyasana:

It provides benefits to sufferers of bronchial asthma and Diabetes Mellitus.

Bhujangasana:
This exercise is good for developing the ligaments of the back and beneficial for the sufferers of backache. It also benefits those with cough and respiratory disease, besides ridding the body of fat or adipose tissue around the abdomen.

Dhanurasana:

This exercise is meant for the relief of stomach disorders and to improve digestion.

Shirsasana:

This exercise, which culminates in a headstand, enhances blood supply to the brain, besides providing a high level of conditioning to the body. It stimulates the thyroid and pituitary glands and is good for relieving a condition known as orchitis, as well as dysfunction connected with virility. It enhances blood flow to the brain and so benefits all brain functions. But it is not to be practiced by people suffering from high blood pressure, otitis media and eye diseases.

Shavasana:

It is good for relieving alleviated levels of blood pressure, inducing sleep and maintaining a tranquil state of mind, and creating a sense of peace.

Vajrasana:
It provides the benefits of relieving stiffness in the knees and legs and in relieving oedema.

Hansasana:
It improves digestion, relieve constipation and stimulates the pancrease, this exercise helps the wrist joints to relax and strengthens the arms.

Mayurasana:

This exercise promates abdominal secretions, relieves indigestion and digestive disorders and conditions the muscles of the abdomen.

Pavanamuktasana:

It relieve constipation and digestive complications.

Sputa Vajrasana:

This exercise brings relief to stiffness and pain in the back and the joints.

Chakrasana:
This serves to stimulate the nervous system, and also provides benefits for conditions of asthma, constipation and diabetes. But it should not to be practiced by people suffering from stomach ulcers, slipped discs and heart disease.

Swasthikasana:

This helps the lower limbs to shed fat while removing stiffness in them. It is also good for the stimulation of the circulatory system and the mind.

Bhadrasana:

It shapes the thighs and is beneficial for the bladder and the genitor-urinary system.

Simhasana:
This is an exercise for the throat, the salivary glands and for sufferers of tonsillitis.

Siddhasana:
It is a classic pose for meditation adopted by multitudes of sages over the years.

Kukkutasana:
It is helpful for those suffering from constipation and retention of urine.

Gomukhasana:

This exercise is beneficial for the spinal cord, in treatment for abdominal disease and it aids in digestion.

Facets of Yoga (Samadhi):

This is the eighth facet of Yoga, enabling the practitioner to reach a state from which salvation is possible. This is the ultimate objective of the practice of Yoga. Samadhi can take two forms:

Samprajnata Samadhi: Samadhi achieved by spurning attachments to the material world is called Savikalpa or Samprajnata Samadhi.

Asamprajnata Samadhi: It is the point of conclusion, when the mind dissociates from the material world, all the afflictions vanish along with image, sight and senses.

Classification of Yoga:

There are a number of ways of developing consciousness. All are Yoga of one sort or another. They may be classified as:

1.   Jnanayoga: Attaining realization through knowledge.

2.   Karmayoga: Attaining realization through action.

3.   Bhaktiyoga: Attaining realization through devotion.

4.   Mantrayoga: Attaining realization through Mantra.

5.   Rajayoga: Attaining realization through meditation.

6.   Hathayoga: Attaining realization through practice and meditation.

Thus, with Yoga, both mental efficiency and activity improve. Yoga preserves and protects health by producing antibodies in the blood and by regulating the mind.

Yoga Healing

Yoga is an ancient philosophy and practice of health and well-being. Thousands of years ago when Yoga was first conceived and practiced, people led physically active lives by necessity. There were no cars, no washing machines, microwave ovens, plumbing systems, etc. The routine of daily life provided people with all of the exercise they needed. It was in this physically demanding world that Yoga originated, not to give people more physical exercise, but as a system of healing with special emphasis on the mind. Today, most people identify Yoga only with āsana, the physical practice of Yoga, but āsana is just one of many tools used for healing the individual. In the Yogasūtra of Patañjali, widely acknowledged as the authoritative text on Yoga, only three of the 195 sūtras mention āsana. The rest of the text discusses the other tools of Yoga, including conscious breathing, meditation, lifestyle and diet changes, visualization, and the use of sound, to name only a few. These tools address all dimensions of the human system: body, breath, mind, personality, and emotions. Four basic principles underlie the teachings and practices of Yoga's healing system:

1) The human system is a holistic entity. It is comprised of different dimensions that are interrelated and inseparable from each other. The health or sickness of any single dimension affects the other dimensions, and vice-versa.

2) Each individual is unique. For this reason, each person's problems must be approached in a manner that addresses the unique needs of that individual. There is no "one-size-fits-all" pill in Yoga.

3) Yoga is self-empowering; the student is her own healer. The teacher can offer direction and give a healing practice, but it is up to the student to do the practice. Unlike other healing modalities, such as surgery or massage, in Yoga the student is empowered and required to participate in her own healing.

4) The quality and state of a person's mind is crucial to healing. If the student maintains a positive state of mind, then healing takes place more quickly. If the student's attitude is negative, then healing may take longer. The yogic path to holistic well-being, therefore, is both extremely comprehensive and highly specific to each person. Yoga does not treat specific diseases or specific symptoms; as stated earlier, it treats the individual and his entire human system: the physical body, the breathing body, the mind, the personality, and the emotions.

One model of healing offered in the Taittirīya-Upaniṣad and used in Yoga is the pañcamaya model. Pañca means "five," and maya indicates "something that is all-pervading." According to this model, the human system is multidimensional— we are not just our physical body, for example. Rather, the human system is comprised of five interconnected and interpenetrating dimensions. Moving from the most gross to the most subtle dimension, they are: the physical body, the breath, the intellect, the personality, and the emotions. Some of the many commentators on the Taittirīya-Upaniṣad have used the word kośa to describe these aspects, but this word is misleading, because it gives the impression that each dimension exists separately from the others. The imagery often used to demonstrate the concept of kośa is the layers of an onion that may be peeled away from each other. The pañcamaya model implies something quite different, however: that these five dimensions are all present, all the time, in each part of the human system, even in each cell of the body. They cannot be "peeled" apart; they are inseparable from each other. What happens on one level or dimension of the human system, therefore, affects the others.Because each dimension is connected to the others so profoundly, it is possible to influence problems in one dimension by working on the other dimensions. For example, conscious breathing with an emphasis on exhalation often provides relief to people who suffer from insomnia. Having offered this example, it is important to note that it is impossible to conclusively universalize the application of a single technique. There is no one-size-fits-all solution to any problem. How a sickness affects me will be different from how it affects another person. Our minds, personalities, attitudes, emotions, and bodies are so different that each of us will require a different solution, even though we may be suffering from seemingly similar problems. Recently, a married couple came to the Krishnamacharya Yoga Mandiram (KYM) seeking help for similar problems: they were both depressed and overweight. Both husband and wife are the same age and work in the same profession. They also shared a similar diet and lifestyle. The reasons for the husband's depression and weight gain, however, were quite different from those of the wife. The wife was depressed because she was overweight, while the man was overweight because he was depressed and had begun drinking too much. We offered the wife practices to reduce her weight, and once she began to notice the effects of this practice, she started to recover from her depression. We gave the husband practices to calm him and reduce his stress, and as a result he stopped drinking, changed his eating habits, and began to lose weight. So although both husband and wife suffered from similar problems, we offered different practices to each of them. The type of practice offered was mandated by each patient's unique needs, not by one-size-fits-all treatment for weight loss and depression. In addition, Yoga teaches us that we do not need to address all at once every problem from which patient is suffering. In the case of both patients discussed above, one problem turned out to be the source of the other. We thus addressed the source or root problem first, and when the root problem was treated, this alleviated the symptoms. In the case of the wife, the root problem was associated with her weight gain and the symptom was depression. In the case of the husband, the root problem was depression and a symptom was weight gain. In both cases, treating one dimension of the patient's system affected other dimensions. Illness, whether it is cancer or depression or a minor backache, does not draw a line between the physical body and the other four dimensions of the human system. If one is affected, the other dimensions are affected. For example, when someone gets angry (emotional dimension), the whole system changes as a single unit: the face reddens and the muscles tense (physical dimension), the breath becomes short, shallow, and rapid (breath dimension), mental attitudes become negative (intellectual dimension), and communication becomes very aggressive (personality dimension). It is also true that illness may manifest most prominently in one dimension: for example, as backache in the physical dimension, or as depression in the emotional dimension. This does not necessarily mean, however, that the root cause of the ailment is in the same dimension. A backache is not necessarily entirely physical (or even primarily physical for that matter), nor is depression entirely emotional. It also does not imply that there is only one cause for the ailment. There may be multiple causes spread over multiple dimensions, and these causes may be related or unrelated: it depends on the individual person, and every person is different.

The Role of the Mind
The mind plays a central role in the healing process. Mind is present in all of our activities; without mind we would not be able to perform any conscious activity— lift a finger, read a book, drive a car, turn a cartwheel, react calmly in a negative situation, etc. The state of our mind greatly influences the quality of our actions. When we are anxious because we are running late to work, we rush around, and that "rushing" quality is evident in all of our actions: from the way we drive the car, to the impatient tone we use when addressing the parking lot attendant who takes too long to give us our ticket. When our state of mind changes, our whole human system changes with it. This is why almost anyone can do Yoga: the only requirement is an active mind. If a person is able to pay attention and is willing to try various practices, he or she does not have to be able to move the physical body at all in order to practice. Only the ability to focus and discipline the mind is essential to healing through Yoga. By changing the quality of our state of mind, we can transform ourselves in a profound and positive way. Steve, a student of mine who lives in Australia, suffered a stroke a few years ago. He woke up in the hospital unable to move the left side of his body,

and his speech and memory were severely impaired. Doctors arranged for him to be treated by a physical therapist, a speech therapist, and a psychologist, as well as by an acupuncturist. After some time had passed with little progress, a friend suggested Steve try working with a Yoga teacher. Although, being partially paralyzed, Steve could not do āsana, it did not mean he could not practice Yoga. His teacher introduced some basic breathing practices and then visualization techniques. She asked Steve to visualize the breath moving to the left side of his body while inhaling and moving from the left side of the body outward while exhaling. This is just one of many visualization techniques Steve's teacher practiced with him, and over time they dramatically influenced his condition. Not long after he began these Yoga sessions, to the amazement of his doctors (and Steve himself), he was able to make small movements with his left hand and leg. After two years, Steve had recovered all of his lost mobility and speech, and he was able to return to his job full time and continue with his life as before.

Healing vs. Curing
At this point, it is important to draw a distinction between healing and curing. In the case of a presently incurable disease like AIDS, where there is little or no hope of recovery despite advanced medical treatment, Yoga's healing model still offers valuable tools. Yoga may not be able to cure a disease like AIDS, but it can still heal the individual by bringing about a positive

change in attitude and quality of life. For example, one of my students in Europe is HIV-positive. Before he started practicing Yoga, he was so depressed that he spent most days in bed doing nothing. After taking a few Yoga classes, however, he became more interested in chanting than in focusing on his disease and spending the day in bed. Gradually, through his āsana and chanting practices, he became interested in Sanskrit, and he is now studying Sanskrit very seriously. He also is taking music classes in order to develop his voice. This is healing: a change in mind, in perception, in attitude. Many conditions tend not to be curable—those with certain illnesses may not be able to live life as they did before the onset of the illness. Yoga, however, can help them make the most of their situation, whatever their state of health, and live a happy, productive life. Yoga makes this possible because the focus of Yoga therapy is healing, which is not the same as curing. Healing implies a method of treatment that is holistic. Curing, on the other hand, implies a method of treatment focused on eradicating illness in one dimension of the human system, typically in the physical body. Whereas the potential of a "cure" may be limited, Yoga offers countless healing and therapeutic options. The lack of a definitive cure for an illness does not mean there can be no healing for the individual. When such healing occurs, mental, emotional, and physical suffering are alleviated, and the patient's quality of life improves. These improvements also may contribute to an increase in the patient's life expectancy. Beyond its holistic, individualized approach to healing, there are additional advantages to Yoga that set it apart from other therapeutic practices. One of these advantages is its self-empowering nature. Yoga engages the student in the healing process. Rather than being a passive recipient of treatment, the student plays an active role in her journey toward health and is primarily responsible for her recovery. The role of the teacher becomes that of a guide directing the student to the tools for recovery and teaching the student how to implement them. The teacher offers the student healing, but cannot do the healing for him or her; the student must commit to the healing process and actively follow the Yoga therapist's instructions. It is the role of the student/patient to practice diligently according to these instructions, observe changes, and report the changes to the teacher. The healing thus comes from within the student, rather than from an outside source. This requirement that the student/patient exercise his or her will in the healing process is deliberate. Medicine has the power in many cases to heal a physical disease and alleviate some psychological disorders, but it is not always effective, as, for example, in the case of paralysis, cancer, or Down syndrome. In addition, it can be argued that a purely medical approach is far less effective in healing the emotional, intellectual, and personality layers of the human system. Where a pill or even surgery may fail, the will, i.e., the focused and deliberate exercise and retraining of the mental muscles, may prove successful. Yoga is, at its root, a science of the mind a philosophy of healing through the conscious focusing of the mind. Bringing both methods together—the Western and the yogic—with one model supporting and complementing the other in an integrated, thoughtfully negotiated plan of treatment, can provide the opportunity for even deeper healing for the patient. For the healing process to move forward, there are a few conditions that must be met. First, the student's mind must be in a state to listen to and understand instructions. For example, if someone is a drug addict and is unwilling or unable to stop taking drugs, he is not ready for Yoga. The mind is not active in such a case, but rather is captive to the drug and will not be responsive to instruction. At the KYM, we never ask people to stop doing anything—the practice leads them to that point, if they follow it. If a person is for some reason incapable of actively receiving and following simple instructions, he or she cannot be helped by Yoga. In addition, for treatment to be completely successful, the student must have full confidence and trust in the healer. This combination of confidence and trust, or faith, is another key element in the healing art of Yoga. This confidence and trust between student and healer provide part of the student's motivation to commit to and complete the healing process. This commitment comes from both sides: the teacher commits to the student, and the student commits to the teacher and to the practice of Yoga. A trust relationship is built over the course of the treatment. Its foundation is the structure of the treatment itself, proceeding from the gross to the subtle, the simple to the complex, moving forward step by step. The trust relationship between the healer and the student is built in the same manner, step by step. There is never any movement into more subtle, deep- seated issues until the student is ready. Only the teacher who knows her student as a unique, complex individual, and not just as a dysfunction, disorder, or disease, can know when this point has been reached. In other words, according to the ancient Yoga masters, only a teacher who cultivates the qualities of a healer will be able to build, maintain, and nurture the kind of trust-based, patient-teacher relationship necessary for Yoga therapy to progress successfully. The essential qualities of a healer are presented below.

Vaidya Lakṣaṇa: The Qualities of a Healer Not everyone can become a healer. Collecting information about the healing process from books and workshops is not necessarily going to bring about the transformation. It is not solely a matter of knowledge—even if a person studies for years, he or she may not become a great healer. The ancient masters spoke of the qualities a person must possess in order to be a competent, effective healer. There are a few people who are born possessing all of these qualities, but most who want to be a healer must actively cultivate them.

Jñāni: One who is wise. A teacher must be knowledgeable and wise. She must know what the sickness is and how to help the student. Wisdom also implies knowledge of one's own limitations. If a healer does not know how to treat a student, he must know where to direct that student, so that the student can receive the appropriate treatment.

Mauni: One who has disciplined communication. A teacher must be able to communicate clearly and effectively. This is crucial to the healing process. Problems can arise if a teacher has poor communication skills. The teacher's speech also must be tailored to the student's ability to hear. A teacher must always reflect carefully before speaking and acting.

Jitātmavān: One who has self-control. A healer must have self-control and be able to maintain self-control throughout the healing process. She must remain firm and detached, retaining presence of mind while also being empathetic. A teacher must never exploit a student or abuse the teacher-student relationship in any manner.

Dāta: One who is generous. A teacher should be generous in many ways: with words, with time, with healing, with his heart. His generosity nourishes self- healing in the student. On the other hand, if a teacher is not generous with his care, healing will not take place. Dāta is related to aparigrahi, the next ⍰uality.

Aparigrahi: One who is modest. While a teacher must be generous, she herself should not accept favors or gifts from a student. Appropriate compensation is one thing, but how do we determine what is appropriate and what is inappropriate? It is the duty of the teacher to refuse what is more than appropriate, even when the student freely offers more. When a teacher accepts gifts or favors that are not appropriate to the relationship, the dynamic between the student and teacher changes, and clarity and trust may be lost. On the other hand, a teacher may perform a favor for the student when appropriate.

Dharma rakṣaka: One who is ethical. In this context, dharma refers to a set of values or ethics, and rakṣaka means "one who protects or upholds." A teacher should be a dharma rakṣaka: a person who respects and practices the ethics of the healing system. In other words, the behavior of the healer is important. Healing takes place within the context of a relationship between a healer and a student, so how the healer behaves has a direct bearing on that relationship and, by extension, on the health of the student. This is not a trivial matter. If a teacher is not a living example of what he teachers, how can he expect the student to respect and follow his instructions?

Sthitadhī: One who has a stable and focused mind. A healer must have a stable and focused mind— Yoga heals through the focusing of the mind. A healer who is not already stable and focused in her own mind will not be able to help cultivate that quality in another. In addition, a teacher who is not stable is likely to project her own problems onto the student.

Satyaparah: One who is honest. The teacher must always interact with the student in an honest way and speak the truth. This does not mean the teacher must necessarily speak all the truth all at once; this depends on the student and his situation, and what part of the truth—all or just a portion—the student is ready to hear. Sometimes the truth is painful and may harm the student or drive him or her away, so the teacher must be sensitive to the student's situation, know what the student is able to hear, and know how to communicate with him appropriately.

Śraddhāvan: One who is confident or has conviction. The teacher must have conviction that the treatment will work and convey that confidence to the student. This cannot be a false confidence: both teacher and student must be convinced of and have confidence in the treatment in order for it to work.

Sampradāya sevaka: One who is committed to a lineage. Sampradāya means "lineage." Each tradition has its own approach to healing and its own way of describing the healing process, and the teacher must be consistent and clear about which lineage she follows. If she is not, she risks generating confusion and distrust between her and her student. In addition, mixing and matching one lineage with another may dilute the efficacy of the practice. If we teach something from another lineage that conflicts with what has already been established in our practice, it weakens the practice's legitimacy.

In other words, a lineage's practices are built upon the specific theoretical foundations of that lineage. Thus, although we may encounter many of the same terms and concepts across lineages, these terms and concepts will vary in subtle and not-so-subtle ways, depending on how a particular lineage interprets them. Such differences are even more pronounced when we look at culturally distinct systems of healing like Chinese medicine and Āyurveda. Even more importantly, a teacher who respects his lineage can always refer back to his teacher when he runs into a roadblock when working with a student. He will always have a tradition to turn to for guidance. In this way, the sampradāya provides invaluable support to the healer. Even within a lineage, there are still times when a teacher wanders from his path, with negative conseᵠuences for his students. We see this happening nowadays. In such a situation, it is the sampradāya that stands behind the student and protects her from the teacher. It is also the sampradāya that sets rules to rehabilitate the teacher. This is another reason why it is so crucial for a student to belong to and serve a tradition of teachers. Unless there is accountability, it is difficult to set and implement clear boundaries in the student-teacher relationship. Let me also say that there is no single path that is suitable for everyone and that can heal every problem. Thus, if as a healer you find you need to access help outside your lineage, send your student to someone you respect and let go of that part of the healing process. Work with what you know. Work with what you can do, with what you can heal.

How Yoga Defines Illness The ancient.

 Yoga masters defined disease or sickness in a specific way based on their holistic view of how our whole human system functions. In order to understand how Yoga heals and make effective use of the tools it offers us for healing, we need to understand the ancient masters' conception. The Yoga masters identified three distinct types of illness, then further differentiated them by classifying them based on the causes(s) and severity of the illness

First, we will look at the three general types of illness as defined by the Yoga masters.

Duḥkham
The Sanskrit word duḥkham usually refers to emotional suffering, but duḥkham is felt on other levels as well. Duḥkham derives from the Sanskrit duh, which means "constriction" and kham, which refers to the space in our heart considered to be in the center of our chest. Duḥkham is thus literally the constricting, tightening, or closing of the space of our heart. The opposite of duḥkham is sukham, or openness in the space of our heart, an expansion of that space.

Roga
Roga refers to discomfort and/or unease that stems from being in a situation in which we do not wish to be.

Vyādhi
Vyādhi has many meanings, but in this context it refers to an imbalance occurring in the three aspects of our physical system: dhātu, rasa, and kāraṇa.

Dhātu refers to the aspects of our system that give form to and sustain the body, such as bones, muscles, and skin. Examples of dhātu imbalance include broken bones, one leg longer than the other, one arm stronger than the other, etc.

Rasa refers to the liquids of the body, such as saliva, blood, tears, menstrual fluid, etc. Examples of rasa imbalance include dry eyes, dry throat, and anemia.

 Kāraṇa refers to our senses, including the mind, eyesight, hearing, smell, taste, and touch. Examples of kāraṇa imbalance are blindness, deafness, and sinus problems. The word vyādhi also can be derived from the Sanskrit vi, meaning "disconnected," and ādhi, meaning "inner consciousness." When we are in a state of vyādhi, we are in a state of illness—we are imbalanced in the three aspects of our human system. This imbalance draws our attention outward: the mind becomes distracted, attaching itself to the pain, discomfort, or disease generated by the physical imbalance. In our distraction, in our imbalanced state, we lose the connection to our stable, balanced core, or inner consciousness.

CHAPTER TEN

Classifications of Disease

Yoga further classifies disease or illness based on the cause and also on the severity or manageability.

1.   Cause
What is the cause of my illness? In other words, who is responsible for my illness?

Ādhyātmika: Myself. I am the cause. For example, a person develops asthma because of her smoking habit. Ādhibhautika: Someone else or an outside cause is responsible: for example, a woman who has contracted HIV or a sexually transmitted disease from her husband, or a person suffering from a dog bite (unless, of course, the person provoked the dog, and then this would be a case of ādhyātmika). In both cases, the individual in question is not responsible for her illness, but someone or something else is.

Ādhidaivika: Divine force is responsible. In other words, something out of our control is the cause:

for example, trauma caused by an earthquake or certain kinds of birth defects.
It is important to know the cause of a sickness, because it influences the course of treatment. The cause of an illness might be just one of the above-mentioned causes or a combination of any two or all three.

2. Severity and Manageability

Susādhya: Easily healed. Minor back pain is an example.

Dussādhya: Not so easily healed. Healing is possible, but with some difficulty. Considerable time and effort will be required, but the situation is not impossible.

Asādhya: Impossible. Some sicknesses (and here we are referring only to the sickness/disease itself, and not to the whole person) are impossible to heal: presently AIDS and mental retardation are examples in this category.

Yāpya: Manageable, even though it cannot be cured. Even though this sickness cannot be removed from the system, it can still be managed in a way that does not worsen it and that may even result in remission. Examples include asthma, AIDS, and mental retardation. I have listed the latter two again on purpose, to emphasize the importance of treating the human system as a whole and each person as a distinct, complex individual. AIDS may presently be an incurable disease, but the person with AIDS can still be healed and the incurable disease managed through readily available AIDS medication. Whether healing will occur after an individualized treatment has been prescribed depends, ultimately, on the person and his or her commitment to the healing process. Two people with the same "easy" sickness may not come through the healing process successfully. One may succeed quickly, while the other may heal much more slowly, or possibly not at all, depending on his or her level of commitment to the healing process.

How the Yoga Therapist Approaches Healing

Step 1: Heyam: Recognizing the Need for Help

The very first step in the healing process actually belongs to the patient, who must recognize that he is in trouble and needs help, and then must seek help. The recognition that we need help is called heyam. Unless a person recognizes that he or she is in trouble, the healing process cannot begin. This recognition happens as a result of familiarity with the symptoms of suffering.

According to Patañjali''s Yogasūtra (YS I-31), suffering expresses itself in four ways:

1. Emotional state: When we become sick, our emotional patterns change, which is another way of saying that our emotions mirror our situation. When we are sad or angry or unhappy, we need to recognize this, admit it, and ask why.

2. Negative mental attitudes: We may become very pessimistic or negative, or begin to find fault in ourselves or others, or in a situation. The mind is not still, but rather is constantly fluctuating.

3. Physiological changes in the body: There may be changes in bodily patterns. For example, the body temperature may change, hair may begin to fall out, the breath may smell bad, dark circles may form around the eyes, we may have digestion or elimination problems, etc.

4. Breathing pattern: The normal breath is long and smooth, but if it becomes short or labored or very heavy, then we know

something is wrong. The human system is, of course, a single whole, and often times we will experience more than one symptom; that is, the different dimensions of our human system will express suffering in different ways.

Step 2: Hetu: Identifying the Causes of Duḥkham, or Suffering

What causes a person to suffer? We know from experience that nothing happens without a cause. If we are suffering, our suffering must also have a cause. In order to heal suffering, the teacher must know and understand the causes of suffering. Some of the causes of suffering are:

Pariṇāma: Change. We suffer because there has been a change, either outside of us or within us. Even a simple change in the weather can trigger allergies, physical discomfort, colds, etc. Another example would be a change in diet. If I travel to another country and cannot eat the food I am used to eating, I suffer. In addition, as I grow older, my body's nutritional needs change, and if I do not temper my eating habits appropriately, I will suffer.

Tāpa: Excessive thirst. Sometimes we have an excessive thirst for certain things like food, sex, alcohol, drugs, etc. Such "thirst" may elevate to an addiction and even to illness. Illness or a negative pattern of behavior may also result when the thirst is not ꞯuenched.

Saṁskāra: Our patterns, habits, and other automatic behaviors. A habit may be appropriate in one context, but not appropriate in another. When you visit England, if you continue to drive on the right side of the road, as is your habit, you will suffer. Habits may also result from experience. For example, after a series of bad luck events, we may get into a habit of negative thinking and see all new situations in a negative light. The problem with automatic behaviors is that we do not think, we just act "automatically," and how we act may or may not be appropriate to the situation. If it is not appropriate, we will certainly suffer.

Asatsaṅga: Inappropriate association or company. The company you keep and the relationships you maintain (social, familial, professional, etc.) are important because they influence you. There is an English adage that illustrates this point very well: if you lie down with dogs you are bound to get fleas.

Asatmya indriya saṁyoga: The linking of the senses to something inappropriate or abusive. In this situation, you can suffer from too much exposure or from underexposure. For example, excessive television viewing and video-game playing or long-term exposure to loud music will certainly causes problems for us over time, especially later in life. Anything, even Yoga, can be overdone.

Ayutka svātmika gauravam: Inappropriate self-esteem. This can mean either excessive ego or lack of self-esteem. There are many obvious examples of how people suffer because of lack of self-esteem or because of excessive ego.

Vāta prakopa: Literally, "angry wind." Anything we do that agitates the breath causes us to suffer. Breathing is central to life, and if we allow the breath to become agitated, the breath will retaliate and cause suffering. This suffering can take the form of bodily twitches or trembling, yawning, flatulence, indigestion, dry skin, bowel and urinary disorders, and even fertility problems. In some of the ancient texts, as well as Āyurvedic texts, there is considerable space devoted to the different kinds of illnesses triggered by Vāta prakopa.

Ayutka āhāra: Inappropriate food or eating habits. This includes what a person eats, as well as how he or she eats—how much, in what way, at what time, where, and with whom.

Ayutka vihāra: Inappropriate lifestyle. This refers to sleeping and exercise habits, where a person lives, who the person lives with, the workplace and work habits, extracurricular activities, etc.

Janmaja: Congenital disorders. These are problems present at birth. Sometimes we see children born with blindness or who are HIV-positive. They are born with their illness, and they cannot be blamed for it.

Īśvara saṁkalpa: Divine will. An example would be a person hit by lightning. There is no explanation for why this should happen, except that it was a random act of nature or "Divine Will." Some may argue that this is a result of karma, but the point here is that the cause is unseen. It is important to note that these categories are not rigidly distinct. They will overlap on many occasions. It should also be noted that this list covers the most important causes, but there are others as well. As healers, we must develop the ability to observe, to be able to look at all the different dimensions of a person and to know what to look for. A healer must know not only what to observe (symptoms), but also how to observe. In Yoga, there are three methods of observation.

The Three Methods of Observation

Darśaṇam: Observation through the medium of the senses. This refers to what we see, smell, hear. Is the student's voice weak or strong? Do I smell bad breath? Do I see drooping shoulders and a collapsed chest? We might also ask the patient to perform a physical posture or two as part of this observation process.

Sparśanam: Observation through touch. This includes such things as taking the temperature or pulse, or feeling the shoulder and neck as a way to check for muscle tightness. When using this method of observation, we should always ask patients if it is okay to touch them before doing so.

Praśnam: Interaction and dialogue. This refers to talking with the student and observing how he or she responds to questions. Do not always take a verbal response at face value. How the patient responds can often tell you much more than what was actually said. Sometimes the truth resides in what a person does not say. The teacher should be adept at utilizing all of the observation methods at once and integrating them in a manner that fits the needs of the unique situation. In other words, the person you are healing is always more important than any checklist of techniques. The unique needs of the student should guide your choices. You are healing an individual, not fulfilling the requirements of any generic, institutional checklist or form.

Continuing with the healing model from Patañjali's Yogasūtra, we now need to decide what we want to accomplish in the healing process. Healers create practices that are designed to address illness and its causes, so it is important to know where we are starting from in the healing process. By the same token, it is equally important to know what the desired result of the healing process is: if we do not know where we are going, how can we decide how to get there? A healer must carefully choose and prioritize reasonable goals for the healing process. Let us therefore discuss some ideas regarding health and determine what we are trying to achieve.

Step 3: Hānam: The Five Elements of Health and Prioritizing Health Goals for Healing
It is important to remember that when someone is sick, the symptoms do not manifest in the physical body only. Whatever the cause, the illness also will affect other areas of the student's life. We thus need to look at all the things that are happening in the student's life, decide what the priorities are in the healing process, and address the priorities first. The five elements of health, presented below, are all possible goals, or hānam, for the healing process. Samatvam: Balance and harmony in the human system. Examples include eyes that are neither dry nor watery; an appropriate, balanced alignment of the body; clear sinuses; efficient, regular digestion and elimination; etc. We look for this quality especially in reference to dhātu, rasa, and kāraṇa.

Arogyam: No "roga," or no dis-ease. There is no anxiety or discomfort in one's situation.

Sthairyam: Stability. This refers to stability of mind, body, energy, emotions, etc. Ideally, an individual daily has the same amount of energy, the same stability and focus of mind, a balanced emotional state, etc.

Dvandva sahanam: The ability to remain undisturbed by extremes (of weather, of circumstances, of emotion, etc.). If it is extremely cold, I am not affected, for example, by this extreme in temperature. I, of course, need to put on a jacket, but this does not agitate me. Responding in a balanced way to shocking news is also dvandva sahanam.

Indriya nigraha: Literally, "holding the senses." A healthy person is someone who has their senses under control, who can direct them or rein them in at will. In such a case, the senses obey the person rather than drawing the person here and there in pursuit of whatever catches the senses' fancy. Sickness results when the senses dominate us, as in the case of any addiction: drugs, food, shopping, sex, video-game playing, etc.

In the process of healing, it is not always possible to address the root cause of illness immediately, because the student is not ready. In such cases, we need to choose intermediate goals. Once we have accomplished these intermediate goals, perhaps then the student will be ready to focus on addressing the root cause of the illness. Our goals must be approached in steps, where one step prepares us for the next and healing takes place gradually.

In selecting short-term goals, a decision needs to be made on how to prioritize them, which leads us to the next issue.

The Application of Śamana and Śodhanam

There are two approaches a healer may take when choosing and prioritizing goals:

Śamana: Pacification. When an individual is suffering a great deal, especially emotionally, the best approach to healing is an indirect one: to first pacify the person and stabilize him, rather than addressing the root of the problem immediately. This means that the roots of the problem will probably remain, but the point here is to bring some stability to the patient before doing any deeper work, which, at this juncture, might threaten or even harm the patient. Śamana is the most common starting point for healing work.

Śodhanam: Refinement and cleansing. Śodhanam is the removal of the root of the problem. In some cases, a student's suffering may be due to a specific cause. For example, I may have stress because of my poor lifestyle choices. We may keep pacifying our stress using certain pacification methods. The stress will continue to exist, however, until the root of the problem, which in this case is the unhealthy life style, is addressed. To address the root cause of the problem is śodhanam. A healer does not have to begin with śamana and end with śodhanam. Every decision, every choice, every step in the healing process is based on the healer's observations and interactions with and knowledge of the individual person. One student may be safely and successfully helped using a śodhanam approach from the outset. Śodhanam often provokes a strong reaction in people, however, so for many it is best if the healer initially adopts a śamana approach. Then, as the healing progresses, the focus can gradually be turned to the root problem.

Śamana may thus be the short-term goal, while śodhanam would be the long- term one.

A woman in her mid-forties came to our center seeking relief from chronic depression. After working with her, we found that the cause of her chronic depression was the poor relationship between her and her husband. The strain in their relationship was caused by some choices the woman had made, but she was not able to look at her own issues right away. She needed to be pacified first, and so this is the method we used with her. Once we had worked with her for a while in this way, she became more calm and stable and was able to look at her own choices and resolve her relationship issues. If we had chosen to confront this patient immediately with her problems, she probably would not have been receptive and might even have abandoned the healing process. This is why a healer needs to make this crucial choice between śamana and śodhanam. Healing takes time; we can't expect to deal with everything at once. We must first determine what it is we want to accomplish and then we prioritize our goals according to the student's unique needs. We approach the healing process one step at a time in a logical, orderly manner that is always attuned to the needs of the student. Who is going to be practicing is always more important than what technique is used.

Step 4: Upāyam: Finding and Implementing the Tools for Healing
Patañjali presented the concept of Upāyam, or tools, last because

only after we know where we are going, and from where we are starting, can we determine how to proceed. If we decide to go to Los Angeles, California, U.S.A., how we travel would be very different if we set out from San Diego, California, U.S.A., rather than from Chennai, Tamil Nadu, India. Likewise, the tools of healing only make sense in the context of their use; if we don't know what sickness the student is suffering from and how we intend to treat her, how can we choose the appropriate tools for healing? We must choose the tools that will help us accomplish our healing goals. If we are going swimming, we would need a different set of tools than if we were setting out for a hike in the mountains. What good is a surfboard to us in the mountains? By the same logic, just because we have access to a tool does not mean it is an appropriate one for us to use. Once we determine the goals for the student, then we can choose the right tools. The goals determine which tools we use, as well as how we use them in the healing process. Before choosing any Yoga tool, there are several factors the Yoga therapist must consider for each patient in order to evaluate whether a tool will be useful in that patient's healing process, and how the tool may or should be applied. These factors include the following:

Kāla: Time. The healer must take into consideration how much time a person can set aside to practice, that is, how much time he or she can comfortably commit to. We might offer a busy executive a fifteen-minute practice to be done twice each day, while a part-time student might be able to set aside 45 minutes every night for practice. We also should consider what time of day the person would be practicing. We tend, for example, to be more flexible at night than we are first thing in the morning. In addition, some practices are very energizing and thus should not be done in the evening. Time of the year is another aspect to consider. Each person reacts differently to seasonal patterns. Spring may bring on allergies, while winter may bring on sinus problems or depression, etc.

Deśa: Place. Where will the student practice? Is the climate tropical, temperate, cold? Altitude makes a big difference as well. In high altitudes, even a seven- second inhale can be difficult, whereas at sea level up to fourteen seconds may be easy.

Vayah: Age. The prescribed practice must respect the restrictions and distinct needs of the student's age. For example, while a thirty-year-old woman could be expected to sit and meditate on the tip of a candle for fifteen minutes, a nine- year-old boy could not. This is why the ancient masters suggested that the main focus (not the only focus) for youth should be āsana, for middle-aged students prāṇāyāma, and for older people meditation.

Vṛtti: Occupation or profession. If the student's job involves sitting at a desk all day, he or she will probably need a more dynamic practice. A farmer, on the other hand, would probably need a less strenuous practice. A psychologist might benefit most from a practice for his body or a practice that clears the mind between meetings with clients.

Śakti: Power or ability. How much physical, mental, and emotional strength does the person have at any given time? We have to respect the abilities of the person.

Icchā: Interest. What are the student's likes and dislikes? Consistent with the student's interests, we can add a few qualities to the tool so that it motivates the student to practice regularly. For example, if a student has a spiritual interest, perhaps a spiritual ingredient might help motivate practice and help generate a positive attitude about practice. As healers, considering these parameters helps us to evaluate the whole person and his or her needs and abilities, instead of fixating on the disease. We can now look at the tools Yoga offers us for healing the whole person.

Śarīrika Cikitsā: Healing Using the Body

There are three methods of healing that engage the physical body.

1. Āsana

Āsana is the practice of physical postures. Our concern as healers when using the tool of āsana is the pose's function, not its outward form. The Yoga masters classified āsanas into five categories based on their functions. Āsana is utilized primarily for affecting the health and well-being of our physical body, but we must remember that all five dimensions of the human system are interconnected: affect one dimension and all dimensions are affected. The physical dimension is the least subtle of the five. If we cannot connect with our physical body, our "grossest" dimension, how can we possibly connect with our subtler ones? Āsana is thus a good starting point, a place to begin to open oneself to the possibility of connecting with the subtler dimensions of the human system. Beyond certain important, practical physical functions, each type of posture serves additional functions that are more subtle. These are based on another model, consisting of the nāaīs, the cakras, and the kuṇaalinī. For our purposes, however, in this introductory article we will briefly discuss only the physical functions of the postures in each category of āsana.

The five main categories of āsana
Samasthiti: These postures are reference postures. The spine in these postures is erect, or vertical. In other words, all of the important vital points of the spine are in a neutral, healthy alignment. When the spine is in correct position, there is no inter-organ pressure: the body is not collapsing too far forward, compressing the organs and throwing the skeletal structure out of proper alignment, nor is the body leaning too far back or too far to one side or the other, etc., which also puts unnatural stress on the organs of the body and on the various joints. It is in these neutral, erect samasthiti postures that the breath is able to flow most freely and easily, so these postures also serve the function of helping to prepare the student for prāṇāyāma and meditation. By extension, therefore, samasthiti postures also contribute to the process of cultivating a calm and focused mind. Postures in this category include samasthiti and tāaāsana. Śavāsana also is classified as a samasthiti posture, although we are lying on the back in this position, and the spine is thus not technically vertical.Paścimatāna: Paścimatāna literally means "stretching the

back of the body." It is important to note that paścimatāna postures should be done on an exhalation. The natural breath accompaniment to a forward bend is exhalation, because as we bend forward, the chest cavity naturally compresses and becomes smaller, expelling (exhaling) the air from the chest. All āsana movements should begin from the point where the starting breath originates for that particular type of posture. In the case of paścimatāna postures, movement must start from the abdomen, as these postures are done on an exhalation. In some cases, when a student's back is overarched or when the stomach muscles are too tight, we practice paścimatāna postures to correct this tendency. In paścimatāna postures we are drawing the abdomen in and up as we exhale, willfully engaging the abdominal muscles to help counteract any tendency, for example, to overarch in the area of the lower back or sink in the belly. Stretching the body in the opposite direction of the misalignment, we help pull the spine back into a neutral, natural alignment. Examples of paścimatāna postures are paścimatānāsana, uttānāsana, and vajrāsana forward bend (commonly referred to as child's pose).

Pūrvatāna: Pūrvatāna may be translated as "stretching the front of the body." The natural breath accompaniment of a backbend is an inhalation, because as we bend backward, the chest cavity naturally expands and gets larger, drawing (inhaling) air into the chest. As pointed out in the previous section, āsana postures start from where the breath begins in that particular type of posture. In the case of pūrvatāna postures, they begin with inhaling, so the movement should begin from the chest. Typically, the physical function of pūrvatāna postures is to bring back to healthy samasthiti alignment a spine that exhibits a tendency to "slouch." For example, people experiencing depression will often exhibit a distinctive posture: chest and shoulders hunched forward and rounded, collapsing the chest area. To counteract this tendency to slouch, which we also frequently encounter in people who work at a desk all day, we might ask the student to work with postures such as pūrvatānāsana, dvipāda pīṭham, or bhujaṅgāsana.

Parivṛtti: These postures involve twisting the body. They are done on exhalation (the same body/breath principle applies here as described above in paścimatāna postures, and so we begin the movement in these postures from the abdomen). Sometimes the spine is straight on the vertical and lateral axis, but it is not aligned on the axial axis (the spine turns, instead, to one side or the other). For example, we encounter this unnatural axial twist in people who tend to sit at work and talk to customers, while also typing on the computer keyboard, which is usually on the table to the right. The body, in such cases, is held in partially "twisted" position for extended periods each day. Postures like trikoṇāsana and jaṭhara parivṛtti can be used to correct this kind of misalignment and bring the spine back to samasthiti.

Pārśva. These postures involve lateral movement of the spine and can be used when working with an individual whose spine is tilted to one side. An example would be a student's shoulders or hips that are uneven due to a birth defect or certain lifestyle choices. Lateral postures like pārśva koṇāsana, pārśva trikoṇāsana, or godhāpīṭham, are examples of pārśva-type postures. This type of posture may be offered to correct misalignment, bringing back lateral symmetry to the body and promoting healthy, samasthiti alignment. There is also a sixth category of āsana, viparīta (inversions) that was created after the others. In most cases, the oldest texts mention inverted postures only very briefly, or not at all. Some masters classify inversions as viśeṣa (special), as if hinting that these are reserved for a special few who are healthy enough to do them. There are few benefits of inversions that cannot be obtained from an appropriate combination of postures drawn from the original five classifications. Inversions thus should be utilized carefully in the healing process, and only used when necessary and the student is ready for them. Remember, āsana impacts not only the physical dimension of the body, but all of the dimensions of our human system. As an example, when we use pūrvatāna postures to correct a stooped posture (physical dimension) resulting from depression (mental and emotional dimensions), we are affecting not just the physical manifestation of the problem, but also the mental and emotional layers of the problem. Often, when performance of the posture improves, the person is able to breathe better. A smoother, longer, more comfortable breath helps to calm the mind and, by extension, the emotions. For this reason, the principle underlying function of any posture, regardless of which category it belongs to, is bringing the posture as close to samasthiti (the healthiest position) as possible. In this way, working only with the physical body, we are able to bring changes to the mind or even the emotions. Sometimes in applying āsana in healing, we may need to utilize many of the functions of the various categories of āsana. We are not limited to one function. We can create for the student a flowing seＱuence of postures combining the desired functions in a smooth, safe way. In addition, some postures combine effects/functions from more than one category. For example, vīrabhadrāsana combines both pūrvatāna and parivṛtti effects, as we start from a position in which we have to twist the spine to face the front. If a student has physical limitations that prevent her from doing traditional postures, we need to identify the functions of those postures we want to offer and create adaptations that preserve them. If we ask the student to do a posture she is not physically able to do, she will get injured. If there is any doubt about what a student is capable of doing, it is always better to be safe. Finally, we must not forget to offer preparatory and counter-poses for any āsana practice. Proper seＱuencing is essential, as it prevents injury and optimizes the healthy effects of the practice. SeＱuencing is a whole science in itself, and a thorough discussion of it is beyond the scope of this introductory article.

2.   Dravya Upayoga

Dravya upayoga is the application of prepared mediums or certain other materials on the body, in particular, the physical application of oils or pastes. Just as with the practice of āsana, the application of oils for specific physical problems may promote healing beyond the physical level. If a student has a stiff neck and we apply oil to help with the stiffness, we also may see results on other levels. There is a whole science behind this, the exploration of which is beyond the scope of this article.

3. Abhyangam

Because Yoga focuses on supporting self-empowerment in the healing process, massage is not mentioned in the Yoga texts. Massage is, however, a part of Āyurvedic healing practices. T. Krishnamacharya, who was also a master of

Āyurvedic healing, said that a good āsana practice is like a massage without a masseur.

In some cases, when the student is unable to move on his own—when he has suffered a stroke for example—then it may be useful to use some massage techniques to alleviate some issues. Here we are again dealing with a topic that falls outside the scope of this article.

Prāṇa Cikitsā: Healing Using Prāṇa

When prāṇa is moving freely throughout the human system, we function in a normal, healthy manner, but when it is obstructed, there is sickness. We can work directly with prāṇa to remove obstructions and promote healing, but before discussing the latter, we should first examine prāṇa itself. Prāṇa is a complex concept that easily could provide enough material for a separate article. For our purposes here, however, our explanation will be simple and brief. Prāṇa refers to both the breath and to a kind of vital energy, or subtle life force, that is within the body and which animates us. As long as we have prāṇa, we have life. If prāṇa leaves, we die. The ancient yogis identified the close connection between breath and life (if we stop breathing, we die) and connected breathing directly with the vital energy that animates the living body. Every cell of our body, they determined, is imbued with prāṇa, and all prāṇa is the same in terms of origin and substance. The ancient yogis gave specific names to prāṇa residing in different parts of the body, however, and attributed specific functions to each.

Description of the five prāṇas
The Yoga masters divided the body's prāṇa into ten different types, called vāyus (literally, "winds") and attributed different functions to each vāyu. We will briefly present five of the most important vāyus, which are called the mahā vāyu (great vāyu). See Figure 1.

Apāna vāyu: Located in the area below the navel, this vāyu is responsible for the vital functions of elimination, reproduction, and fertility.

Samāna vāyu: Located in the area of the belly around the navel, this vāyu is responsible for digestion.

Prāṇa vāyu: Located in the heart and chest area, this vāyu is responsible for mental functions, thoughts, and emotions. In other words, the ancient Yoga masters believed that the seat of the mind is in the heart, not the head.

Udāna vāyu: Located in the throat region, this vāyu influences communication and expression functions.

Vyāna vāyu: This vāyu is present throughout the human system, but it is specifically responsible for moving prāṇa throughout the body. It also is responsible for functions in those areas not influenced by the other vāyus. It is responsible for movement of the fingers and toes, for example.

Figure 1

If a student is experiencing a problem in a specific area of the body, one of the ways we can address that problem is by prescribing practices that work on the vāyu responsible for that area. The most powerful tool for working with prāna is prānāyāma. Patañjali defines prānāyāma as "conscious breathing" (YS II-49). It is impossible to discuss the application of prānāyāma for specific ailments, because the needs and abilities of the whole person, not just how to treat their ailment, must be considered before prescribing a practice. Generally speaking, however, we can use the exhalation and holding after exhalation to work with the apāna vāyu. Inhalation and holding after inhalation influence the prāna vāyu, and breathing ratios in which the inhalation and exhalation are of equal length influence the samāna vāyu. Another important tool for working with prāna is the set of practices known as bandhas. Bandhas are advanced techniques and should not be used casually or without the guidance of a knowledgeable teacher. If a knife is used correctly, it is a very useful tool, but if used incorrectly it can cause severe damage. Similarly, when utilizing prānāyāma and bandhas, if we force things or apply the wrong breathing ratios, we may agitate whatever problems already exist in the student's system. Additionally, bandhas do not engage automatically (there are a few exceptions where it may happen automatically, such as

234

jālandhara bandha in the posture dvipāda pīṭham). The practitioner must engage bandhas willfully, and this is easier to do in certain postures than in others. The ancient texts that discuss bandhas advise that they be done only in samasthiti postures, i.e., when the spine is straight. Having offered these cautions, generally speaking, we can say that jālandhara bandha will bring attention to the throat region and thus affects the udāna vāyu. Uaaīyāna bandha brings additional attention to the apāna vāyu and to the samāna vāyu, and mūla bandha influences the apāna vāyu. The Yoga masters claimed that as the breath becomes longer and smoother, prāṇa flows more freely throughout the human system. So anything that helps the practitioner to smoothly and comfortably extend breathing is a good tool. A long breath by itself is not enough, however—the breath must be not only long, but also comfortable. If the breath is long and ragged, or if we have to strain to make our breath long, we are working in the wrong direction and will likely aggravate any problem. n addition to the bandhas, techniℚues, including āsana, prāṇāyāma may be combined with other, complementary healing bhāvana (visualization), mudrās, oils, and chanting (adhyayanam). For example, when chanting, we produce sound only while exhaling, so we can use the pronunciation of sounds as a way to help the student extend exhalation. Chanting is a powerful tool for healing imbalances of the udāna vāyu. Beyond this most obvious application, chanting also has the potential to influence all of the vāyus, as each Sanskrit sound resonates at a specific location in the body. Ha, for example, resonates in the throat, while ra resonates in the belly. The Sanskrit sound hra resonates in both. That is why it is absolutely crucial that when chanting in Sanskrit, we pronounce each sound correctly. The meaning of the sounds and words are secondary: it is most important to master the correct pronunciation. It should also be pointed out that chanting is not a musical activity; we do not sing the sounds, we speak them. There is a difference between kīrtan and adhyayanam. Singing the sounds changes them, and since the sound has a specific function in adhyayanam, we do not want to alter it in any way. Other techniques that work on prāṇa are mudrā, or hand gestures, and bhāvana, or visualization. Most mudrās influence the vyāna vāyu, because mudrās require consciously directed movement of the fingers and hands. In order to get our hand to hold the desired shape, we have to concentrate, and this conscious effort stimulates the prāṇa in the area of the hands (vyāna vāyu). If we then move our hands to the chest region, we are directing the focus to the prāṇa vāyu. The point here is that bringing the mind's attention to a particular area of the body stimulates the prāṇa in that area. Mudrā accompanying prāṇāyāma would be one possible way to work with someone with Parkinson's disease, an imbalance in the vyāna vāyus. Bringing one's awareness to these physical actions (the mudrās) with prāṇāyāma focuses and redirects the imbalanced vāyus. For example, we can use the "cin" mudrā (which is joining the index finger with the thumb) during prāṇāyāma. During every breath, the person can be asked to change the finger that links with the thumb. This brings the person's attention to the fingers, and hence facilitates the flow of prāṇa. As the ancient masters said, wherever our attention is, there flows prāṇa. What this practice may do is strengthen the vyāna vāyu, whose weakness may be a cause of the trembling of our hands. As is true for every example used in this article, however, this is merely an illustration, and we must not think of this as a prescriptive way to work with people with Parkinson's. Visualization is another powerful technique for working with prāṇa. When I visualize that I am a mountain or that I am sending the breath to my knee, for example, this is what "happens" during the visualization. And this experience, originating from my visualization, has an affect on me. One of the ways we can use visualization is through intention. In Sanskrit this is known as saṁkalpa: the idea that I am now going to do something, an intention to do something. For example, I might say, "I am now going to work on inhalation to influence the prāṇa dimension of my system, and I am going to do this by putting my hands on my chest and visualizing the inhalation getting longer and longer." As we engage in this visualization process, the system changes and our breath does become longer. Finally, kriyās may also be used to work on prāṇa, but we do not advise that they be used. It is too easy to misuse kriyās, and many Yoga masters have said that the same effects can be achieved in safer manner through the use of prāṇāyāma alone. Indriya Cikitsā: Healing through the Senses. Having discussed the physical body as well as prāṇa, let us move on to an even more subtle level of our human system that can be used for healing: indriyas, or the senses. Before we can discuss the senses as tools for healing in Yoga, however, we need to understand how the ancient yogis understood the role of the senses in our lives. Beyond the pañcamaya model of the human system, there exists an even deeper aspect, which is the foundation of our being. In Yoga, this center of our being is called puruṣa, cit, and drastṛ. These different Sanskrit names indicate the same thing, but emphasize slightly different aspects of it (just as brother, son, and husband all describe "me," yet emphasize different aspects of me). Puruṣa means "one who dwells in the city," cit means "that which is conscious" or "that which cognizes," and drastṛ means "that which perceives." In other words, there is something at the very core of our human system that is conscious, that perceives (or is the source of perception), and that is the master of the human system. This core is fundamentally different from the five dimensions of our human system as presented in the pañcamaya model: the core is "spirit," while the five dimensions are "matter." Although this core is both the source of perception and the source of cognition, it cannot function in the world on its own. It requires a medium through which it can act. That medium is the five dimensions of the human system: body, breath, personality, intellect, and emotions. Through these dimensions, which encompass the senses, puruṣa, or consciousness, functions in the material world.The metaphor traditionally used to illustrate the relationship between the puruṣa and the rest of the human system is that of a lame man and a blind man cooperating in order to live successfully in the world. Puruṣa is the lame man:

puruṣa can see, but cannot walk. The human system (pañcamaya model), including the senses, is the blind man; he can walk, but he cannot see. The blind person carries the lame person on his shoulders; they work together (consciousness and material body) as one, because without each other, they cannot function.   The point at the heart of this metaphor is that body, mind, and senses are tools only. Mind is not the source of cognition: it is merely a tool, a kind of mirror, which reflects cognition. Cognition itself originates from a place other than mind. Of course, the quality of the tools (body, mind, and senses) matters. They must be healthy if we want to live a healthy, balanced, fulfilling life. If the tools are defective, the results of the actions that utilize these tools will be flawed. In other words, if the senses are unhealthy, out of balance, or undisciplined, then puruṣa "has no legs," and its movements in the world will be equally unbalanced, undisciplined, and flawed. As the Yogasūtra says, suffering and sickness are bound to be the result.

What Are the Senses?

According to the Yoga masters, the senses, or indriyas, are a subtle kind of matter that helps puruṣa to function in the world. The ten senses help the puruṣa in two different ways, and thus the masters divided them into two categories: senses that gather information and senses that enable us to act.

Jñāna indriya: Literally, "knowledge senses." Hearing, touching, seeing, tasting, and smelling are the senses that support perception by gathering information about the surrounding world in the form of sound, feel, sight, taste, and smell.

Karma indriya: Literally, "action senses." These senses support our actions and enable us to do things. These action senses underlie a kind of power or capability of the hands, legs, reproduction system, speech, elimination processes, etc. Both types of senses can cause us problems, but in different ways. For example, blurry sight or a diabetic being overcome by temptation and indulging in sweets are examples of jñāna indriya malfunctions. Acting violently or telling lies are examples of karma indriya malfunctions. Since the two sets of senses malfunction in different ways, different practices are suggested to address the problems associated with them.

Indriya Cikitsā: Tools for Disciplining and Healing through
the Senses
To maintain the health of the karma indriyas, Patañjali suggests (in sūtras II-30 to II-45) that we cultivate certain attitudes and behaviors called the yamas and niyamas. These are essentially strategies or disciplines for keeping the senses of action pure and, as a result, healthy. Yamas are rules governing our conduct and interactions with others. They are specific social practices we should follow. For example, if I speak to someone in a way that harms him, I am abusing the sense of communication (speech). If, however, I restrain myself and speak in a way that does not cause harm, I am healing myself, because I am actively taking steps to stop a certain cycle of behavior that causes suffering to myself and others. If someone steals, then he also is creating a certain kind of cycle as well as actively participating in a negative pattern of behavior that will probably cause trouble later on. If

we change our conduct, our behaviors, however, we can change our life. In the Yogasūtra, Patañjali offers five yamas: Ahimsā: Non-harming. Anything that hurts another being should be avoided. This means practicing nonviolence, not only at the physical level, but also the mental and communication levels. In every situation, before acting we should pause and consider the other's position. Satya: Truthfulness. Satya encompasses more than simply speaking the truth. Satya means speaking the truth that is consistent with Ahimsā. This is not just "the truth," but how we speak the truth. Speaking the truth may hurt another, and in such a situation it may be better to say nothing. Satya should not conflict with our efforts to behave with Ahimsā. Asteya: Not stealing. This means not taking something that does not belong to you. Asteya encompasses many different levels: material (for example, money), intellectual (for example, plagiarism), etc. It is nonattachment in word, thought, and action to objects belonging to others. To practice asteya is to refrain from serving only your own interest or harming somebody else's. Brahmacarya: Appropriate sexuality. Brahmacarya is a complex concept, often translated simplistically as "sexual abstinence." Brahmacarya literally means "a person moving toward ultimate truth," and it refers to our responsibilities in different situations and throughout the course of our lifetime. As a husband, my responsibilities are different from those I must fulfill in my role as a teacher or as a student. Since each of these roles is different, although each one is a part of me, it is impossible to generalize about what I must do in any specific situation. It is possible, however, to say that we must act in a way appropriate to our responsibilities in any given situation. In other words, I must uphold my responsibilities in a manner consistent with the hat I am wearing at the time. Aparigraha: Not to receive what you do not deserve. The idea is to not grasp things, not to hold onto or accumulate things, but to take only what is necessary. In other words, do not take advantage of the situation. A doctor receives money for seeing a patient: is it right that he also receives a commission for prescribing certain medicines? A teacher receives a fee for giving instruction, but just because her student, in gratitude, offers her one million dollars, this does not mean the teacher should accept it. Niyamas are personal disciplines, attitudes we should adopt regarding ourselves. There are five niyamas. Śauca: Cleanliness, inside and out. Outer cleanliness refers to the normal routine of personal cleanliness: bathing, brushing our teeth, other grooming practices, etc. Inner cleanliness refers to the healthy functioning of our body, as well as to clarity of mind. Practicing āsana and prāṇāyāma are both means of attending to śauca, as are approaching diet and lifestyle practices with care. Saṅtoṣa: Contentment with what we have. When we have saṅtoṣa, we do not covet what is beyond our resources. Saṅtoṣa encompasses our mental activities, physical efforts, and the way we earn a living. If I am content with what I have, I will be happy and calm. But if I am discontented and agitated, I will not respond appropriately in my relationships, and this is bound to cause problems sooner or later.

Tapas: Cleansing process. Tapas refers to the process of eliminating undesirable elements from all levels of our human system. We have defects, and if we don't correct these defects, we will suffer. Of course, removing unhealthy elements from our life is difficult. Tapas means, literally, "to heat." Just as the impurities are eliminated from iron ore by heating the ore, so too impurities can be removed from our system through intense, concentrated effort. There are many different ways to eliminate rubbish from our system, including refining our eating habits, āsana and prāṇāyāma practice, meditation, etc.

Svādhyāya: Understanding the self results from self-examination. All learning, all reflection, all contact that helps us to learn more about ourselves is svādhyāya. Tapas has no meaning without svādhyāya. How do we identify the defects that need to be removed from our system, or what efforts do we need to undertake to do this? The more I know about myself, the better I am able to identify and then begin to eliminate the unhealthy tendencies in my system. Īśvara praṇidhāna: Acceptance of a higher force. Literally, īśvara praṇidhāna means "to surrender to the Lord." We are not the masters of everything we do: many aspects of life are beyond our control. All we can do is act, and the result of that action depends on many different factors, most of which are beyond our control. The point is to focus on the action, not the result of the action, to pay attention to the quality of our actions and accept whatever may happen. If we do what is right simply because it is right, then we will always have a clear conscious. But if we act in order to achieve a certain result, we may or may not achieve that result, and who knows how we will feel about ourselves afterward. To address problems related to the jñāna indriyas, we offer practices that distract these senses from their habitual patterns and provide them with a healthier focus. Practices and techniques used to discipline the jñāna indriyas are called pratyāhāra, literally, "opposite food " We give the affected sense a food other than its habitual, unhealthy food, so that it no longer seeks the unhealthy option. For example, a student who was suffering from various skin problems approached our center. Through consultation and primary examination, we determined that the woman's skin problems were due to a liver problem. This in turn, we found out, was caused by a very inappropriate eating pattern. The course of action suggested was to put the student on a strict diet and a moderate exercise regime. The discipline of replacing her normal food with a new, healthier diet proved to be a pratyāhāra that saved her from further agony. Over time, through her strict adherence to our dietary suggestions, her problems vanished.Traditionally, problems associated with the jñāna indriyas have been illustrated through the metaphorical image of a chariot pulled by five horses (which signify the five senses). As long as the charioteer maintains control of the horses, the chariot (the body) functions well. But as soon as the horses become undisciplined, the chariot is pulled hither and thither and eventually it is pulled to pieces. In other words, if the senses are allowed to choose their own (often unhealthy) directions, they will pull us along with them. If we can discipline the senses, however, control them and focus them, then the chariot of our body will function well. To discipline the senses is difficult. If we are going to shift the senses away from a habitual focus, we must offer a replacement object or objective. We are thus not actually "withdrawing" the senses from a particular focus: we are deliberately re-focusing the senses on an object or direction of our choice. We are replacing an unhealthy focus with a healthy one. For example, trāṭaka (meditating on a candle flame, which trains the gaze and the mind/thoughts) forces the senses and the mind to go in a particular, chosen direction (the flame). The senses are not allowed to wander aimlessly, but are drawn in the specific direction. Other examples are nāda (cutting off the sight, smell, hearing, and taste and listening only to the heart sound in order to train the hearing to become sharper and more focused), eka rasa āhāra (eating only one particular taste for ten days to stimulate one kind of taste bud, then changing to another taste, thus refining over time the sense of taste), and mauna vrata (a vow of silence to train both the sense of hearing and speech). Each of the tools we have discussed here, yamas, niyamas, and pratyāhāra, has an important element in common: the use of the will. Conscious choice plays a critical role in each of these practices. One way to view it is the following: yama is the practice of conscious thought, niyama is the practice of conscious behavior, and pratyāhāra is the practice of conscious perception. These practices thus will not work unless the student has a strong desire to succeed and is committed wholeheartedly to the practice. Some people react negatively to this kind of self-disciplined practice, and, as in all cases, the healer must observe carefully to see if the practice is causing the student more agitation. If it is, then the approach must be changed.

Manasika Cikitsā: Healing Using the Mind

There are so many different ways to use the mind in healing that we cannot possibly discuss them all here. Moreover, mind clearly plays a central role in all of the tools that we have discussed thus far, not just manasika cikitsā. If we are unable to pay attention, even for short periods of time, we will not be able to practice any of the techniques presented in this article. Practice requires attention. If during my morning āsana practice I am constantly thinking of the tasks waiting for me at work, then I am, for all intents and purposes, already at work, because my mind is preoccupied with work. My body may be going through the motions of trikoṇāsana, but I am not doing my āsana practice, because my mind is engaged in something else. Presented another way: mind is fundamental to all of our activities. Consequently, it is fundamental to any healing process in which we are actively engaged. In fact, we can say that mind is the central tool of healing in Yoga. We could go on here to discuss the role of the duality of the mind in healing and also specific meditation techniques, which are essentially innumerable, but these topics, although important, do not fall within the scope of this article. For our purposes, we need to focus on how mental activities heal the human system.

Bhāvana: The term bhavana derives from the Sanskrit root bhû, meaning "to be." Bhāvana refers to visualization—not just visualization of objects, like the sun or the moon or light, but also of certain attitudes we might desire to cultivate in ourselves, such as compassion or courage or stability. For example, I know I have to attend a meeting with a person with whom I do not get along. If before the meeting I visualize how I will deal clearly and effectively with that person, then when I do see him, there will be a subtle change in how I communicate with him. I change my attitude using visualization, and I thereby change the situation and myself. Visualization also can involve visualizing movements of the body, as in the case presented earlier of the student who had suffered a stroke. The doctors told this young man that he would never be able to move certain areas of his body again. As a practice, his Yoga teacher offered him prāṇāyāma in combination with some visualization, asking him to visualize himself raising the affected arm and leg. Gradually, over time, he regained mobility in the paralyzed areas.

Dhyānam: This term means "meditation." Meditation serves two purposes in the healing process of Yoga. First, meditation helps us to refine our mind, so that we can act in a manner appropriate to the situation in which we find ourselves at any given moment. In this sense, one of the definitions of meditation according to Yoga is "refining the memory." Our past experiences leave impressions on us, and these past impressions influence our current perception, sometimes appropriately, other times inappropriately. When I meet an old friend, I do not just see him, I simultaneously remember some past experiences we had together, remember his face, personality, the emotions he invoked in me, etc. How else would I be able to recognize him in a crowd of people and differentiate him from everyone else I have ever met? Memory is thus very useful to us. On the other hand, past impressions can become so powerful and influential in our behavior that they control our actions. We no longer respond to the actual situation as it is, but instead respond according to our habitual way of thinking, which may not be appropriate to the actual situation. Responding inappropriately can cause suffering for us and for others. Once, when I was in an airplane traveling home to India, I felt a tap on my shoulder and heard a voice, "Hello, Kausthub—how are you?" I turned my head and recognized the person behind me as a schoolmate I had not seen in nearly fifteen years. The moment I saw him, however, rather than greet him with the same politeness he had shown me, I spoke in a rude and rather ugly manner, which shocked us both. I later recalled the issues left unresolved between us since childhood and realized that I needed to resolve these patterns of behavior. These patterns had no value in the present, yet they surfaced as soon as I recognized my schoolmate. I was struck by the power of the patterns that dominate our lives, and I went back and apologized to him. Meditation in this sense means recognizing our automatic behaviors, sorting through them, and creating new ones that are appropriate to the changing situations in our lives. The second important purpose meditation serves in Yoga is related to what happens as a result of our meditation practice. We should think of meditation as a process comprised of three aspects: there is a meditator (a perceiver), there is something that is perceived or meditated upon (an object), and there is the link between the two. Meditation is the process of gradually deepening the relationship between these three aspects.

Step 1: Dhāranā
The first step in the meditation process is for the meditator to choose an object to focus on. This "object" can be a thing or a concept or a word, but it must be something. Meditation here is not making the mind "blank," or nothingness of mind. Meditation is focusing on a specific, chosen object, directing the mind toward that object, and maintaining focus on the object. This is not easy. Choosing an object and staying focused on that object alone requires a great effort of will.

Step2: Dhyānam
If we succeed in focusing our mind in a chosen direction and in maintaining that focus, then gradually the link between the meditator and the object deepens. The link eventually deepens to such an extent that the meditator is aware of only two things: the object she is focused on and the feeling she is perceiving it. Nothing else is perceived only the focus of the mind is perceived. At this point, only the faculties of the mind necessary to perceive and understand the object are operating.

Step 3: Samādhi

If we are able to maintain this link and it continues to deepen, at some point the link between the meditator and the object becomes so strong that even the feeling "I am perceiving" drops away, and there is only the object. It is as though the meditator disappears and only the object exists. The more intense the link becomes, the more we experience the object. Most importantly, as we continue to link with the object, deepening our connection and our experience of the object, we gradually assimilate the qualities of the object of meditation. In other words, we slowly become like the object, and this is how healing occurs as a result of meditation. Consequently, choosing an appropriate and relevant object of focus is crucial. The object must not only be appropriate for the situation, but also for the individual. For example, a teacher might ask a student who lacks the quality of stability, whose mind or relationships or emotions are unstable and unbalanced, to use the image of a mountain as his object of focus. This does not mean, however, that every "unstable" person should meditate on a mountain. If the student has had a bad experience on a mountain, it will be very difficult for that person to focus on one. A mountain, therefore, would be an inappropriate, potentially harmful choice for that student. The student's behavior is the indicator of whether or not a meditation practice is working appropriately. Since the student should be assimilating the qualities of the object, the state of her mind should change, and as the state of her mind changes, so should

250

her behaviors. When there is a positive change in the quality of the mind, the student's life and relationships should improve. This is why we often say that we know whether a person's Yoga is working by the quality of his or her relationships.

Ādhyātmika Cikitsā: Healing from the Core
With ādhyātmika cikitsā, as with indriya cikitsā and manasika cikitsā, we are using more subtle tools than the physical body or even the breath to heal an individual. Ādhyātmika cikitsā is healing using our "core," i.e., the deepest, most subtle layer of who we are. According to the Yoga masters, this core is pure consciousness. There are several tools that may be used with ādhyātmika cikitsā, but we will present only the two most important ones here.

Īśvara Praṇidhāna
This can be interpreted in two ways as it applies to the work of ādhyātmika cikitsā.

Faith
Here, we are not referring only to spiritual or religious faith, although īśvara praṇidhāna encompasses these aspects of faith as well. Faith, in this context, means faith in a higher force, be it God, Nature, or something else. The point is you do not have to believe in God or be engaged in religious practice in order to have faith. When we have faith in something higher than ourselves, whatever this higher force may be, then in times of suffering, we are able to maintain a positive outlook and are less likely to suffer even more from fear, anxiety, and

despair. In this way, faith contributes to our healing. My father and his friend, the late Dr. B. Ramamurthy, who was one of the finest neurosurgeons in the world and the first from India, were once discussing the role of the brain in healing. I was very curious about this subject, particularly about the impact of faith on healing. I asked Dr. Ramamurthy if faith had any value at all in the healing process. "Our body functions on signals sent by the brain," he answered. "If the brain sends a signal to the hand to move, it moves. If the brain sends a signal to the eye to open, it opens. Everything in our body happens based on signals the brain sends. And these signals can be either positive or negative, and this makes a whole difference to how we are and how we function. When we have fear, anxiety, etc., the brain sends negative signals, and this is why we feel the way we feel when [we are] overpowered by such feelings. However, when we have faith or confidence, the brain sends positive [signals] and this is what promotes healing. This is known in medicine as the "placebo effect." Our ancient masters called it śraddhā." few years ago, my father was treating a woman with breast cancer. The woman's doctor was recommending surgery, but the woman was frightened and resistant. When my father expressed his support for the doctor's recommendation, however, she immediately agreed to undergo the surgery. My father assured her before she left that he would be praying for her on the day of the operation.

Just as he had promised, on the morning of the scheduled surgery, my father did some chanting in the sannidhi (a small, sacred space on the grounds of our home) and also made an offering of flowers. Afterward, my father gave the flowers to me and asked me to bring them to his patient at her house. When I reached the woman's house, she was just about to leave for the hospital. Relief softened her face when she saw the flowers in my hands. She knew her teacher had prayed for her; I did not have to explain. The surgery was successful. When the woman met with my father afterward, she related a conversation she had with her doctor just before the operation. The doctor, she told my father, remarked on how calm she was. He said that he had never seen a woman with breast cancer awaiting surgery appear so calm. "I know my teacher has prayed for me," she told the doctor. "So, why should I worry?" This is an example of ādhyātmika cikitsā. The woman knew deep in her heart, in her consciousness, that her teacher was supporting her; she had faith in her teacher, and so she was not agitated. She was at peace, even though in such a situation the mind may bring up all kinds of fears and anxieties. She was, however, not affected by the fluctuations of the mind: her faith was stronger.

....and then

The word yoga is often interpreted as "union" or a method of discipline from the Sanskrit word "yuj" (to yoke or bind). A male

practitioner is called a yogi, a female practitioner, a yogini. The Postures The contemporary western approach to yoga is not based on any particular belief or religion, however Yoga does has its roots in Hinduism and Brahmanism. Yoga was developed by seers or ascetics living primarily in the southern parts of India. The seers observed nature and lived as close as they could to the earth, studying the many aspects of nature, the animals and themselves. By observing and emulating the different postures and habits of the animal kingdom they were able to develop grace, strength and wisdom. It was through these very disciplined lives that the practice of the yoga postures were developed. It was necessary to develop a series of postures to keep the body lithe and able to endure long periods of stillness when in meditation.
The Writings ....